THE 5TH DIMENSION

I am fully, freely, and willingly [...]
of the 5th Dimension.
I know and trust that by fully being in the 5th Dimension, I will
witness Miracles today.
My heart is open and ready to receive the love and intimacy of
God Consciousness.
When fully trusting God in the 5th Dimension, I can hear and
feel and have a shift, and everything in my life is easy
and abundant.
Through the Divine, my gifts are fully awakened today in the
5th Dimension.
I am healed in the 5th Dimension. I feel amazing in the 5th
Dimension.
I love being in the 5th Dimension.
I feel peace, love, and joy in the 5th Dimension.
I am trusting that the negative 3rd Dimensional mind chatter
is quickly overcome by the 5th Dimension.
My mind is automatically focused on the present moment with
no effort required.
My mind is simply a state of being.
I automatically live in the 5th Dimension.
My heart is open in the 5th Dimension.
I am a child of God.

Praise for *Awakening to the Fifth Dimension*

"Kimberly Meredith does an outstanding job of taking readers through a journey of medical healing and personal growth. **This book is destined to become a spiritual classic!**"
—Thomas John, psychic Medium, star of *The Thomas John Experience,* and author of *Never Argue with a Dead Person: True and Unbelievable Stories from the Other Side*

"**Kimberly Meredith is an extraordinary healer, and this is an extraordinary book.** You will learn the dynamics of 5D healing and many techniques you can use immediately to strengthen your immune system and live a healthy, vibrant life."
—John Gray, *New York Times* bestselling author of *Men Are from Mars, Women Are from Venus*

"As a sound healer, I work with audible frequencies and have seen the power that healing music can have. When I first experienced Kimberly Meredith's meditation, I felt the healing energy of the inaudible frequencies that she channels. **Kimberly is a gifted healer, and her teachings help and heal many.**"
—Steven Halpern, pioneering sound healer and Grammy-nominated recording artist

"*Awakening to the Fifth Dimension* is the **ultimate guide to healing**, happiness, and a limitless life."
—Gay Hendricks, bestselling author of *The Big Leap* and *The Genius Zone*

"Now with the advance of the new paradigm in science, remote healing is just as scientifically valid as classical proximal healing. And spiritual healing is the medicine of the future, transcending both space and time. This book testifies to these truths and shows that Kimberly Meredith is the Edgar Cayce of our time. This book will be **your guide to a healthy and wonderful life**."

—Dr. Ervin Laszlo, author of *Science and the Akashic Field*

"Kimberly has a unique ability to sense areas of the body and mind that need healing and to direct appropriate healing energy to those areas. Other famous healers and intuitives, such as Edgar Cayce, gave a great variety of suggestions for healing, but he did not lay hands on, or focus scalar energy, to the many who consulted him. Caroline Myss is a gifted medical intuitive, but she does not provide spiritual healing. Kimberly, though still early in her successful spiritual healing work, **has the potential to become one of the greatest healers and medical intuitives of this century**."

—from the foreword by C. Norman Shealy, M.D., Ph.D., CEO of the International Institute of Holistic Medicine and bestselling coauthor of *The Creation of Health* (with Caroline Myss)

"Full of love and concern for humanity, Kimberly Meredith has given the world a sacred gift. What you have in front of you are miraculous formulas from the unique perspective of a person who has undergone profound transformations. With two near-death experiences and years of trials and tribulations, Kimberly knows that the 5th Dimension is not just a spiritual fantasy, it is a practical manifestation of a happier, healthier, and more abundant way of being. Through her hard work she shares **profound ways of healing** that give us the keys to new realities. Use them and change your life." —Alan Steinfeld, author of *Making Contact* and the producer of New Realities

"This book is profound, with compelling information on how to catapult oneself in the 5th Dimension of healing for both mind and body. Inspiring and uplifting, you will learn to **tap into your full potential. A must-read!**"
—Anita Moorjani, *New York Times* bestselling author of *Dying to Be Me* and *What if* This *is Heaven?*

"I have investigated spiritual healing, paranormal phenomena, and miracle healing as a hobby since I could read. From my direct experience of her work, Kimberly Meredith has the gift of medical mediumship. And she can teach you how to align with the incoming energy of 5D consciousness currently showering the Earth Plane. Her book is a great reminder of where to direct my attention whenever I get knocked down by the material world. I love Kimberly and her work!"
—David "Avocado" Wolfe, nutritionist, author, organic farmer, and adventurer

"I highly recommend this book. In reading this book, you will realize that Kimberly's transformation as she puts it from a 4th Dimensional reality to a 5th Dimensional reality attests that we are far more spiritual and electrical than we are chemical and physical. With this understanding, we can see how to heal and take better care of ourselves. As you read this book, imagine yourself to be Kimberly and **become the spiritual healer that is in you. Be all you can be**." ———Dannion Brinkley, *New York Times* bestselling author of *Saved by the Light*

"'May this book open a door for you . . . a portal into the 5th Dimension way of thinking and living.' This is Kimberly Meredith's invitation to all of us. She offers **simple, practical guidance** into a future filled with unconditional love, grace, honor, joy, and radiant health. I have had the privilege of experiencing Kimberly's gift of healing. She is truly a blessing to the world."

———Catherine Oxenberg, activist, actress, and author of *Captive: A Mother's Crusade to Save Her Daughter from a Terrifying Cult*

"This isn't just a book, but **a transformational companion for self-empowerment** in healing, miracles, and true love. Whether you're just starting on your spiritual journey or a multidimensional master, Kimberly's book will open your heart and mind to a brand-new dimension—one where anything is possible." ———Jessica Origliasso, The Veronicas

AWAKENING TO THE FIFTH DIMENSION

Discovering the Soul's Path to Healing

KIMBERLY MEREDITH

Revolutionary Wisdom from One of the World's
Most Respected Medical Intuitive Healers

ST. MARTIN'S
ESSENTIALS
NEW YORK

First published in the United States by St. Martin's Essentials, an imprint of St. Martin's Publishing Group

AWAKENING TO THE FIFTH DIMENSION. Copyright © 2021 by Kimberly Meredith. All rights reserved. Printed in the United States of America. For information, address St. Martin's Publishing Group, 120 Broadway, New York, NY 10271.

www.stmartins.com

Designed by Steven Seighman

Library of Congress Cataloging-in-Publication Data

Names: Meredith, Kimberly, author.
Title: Awakening to the fifth dimension : discovering the soul's path to healing / Kimberly Meredith.
Description: First edition. | New York : St. Martin's Essentials, 2021. | "Revolutionary wisdom from one of the world's most respected medical intuitive healers."
Identifiers: LCCN 2021015927 | ISBN 9781250780225 (hardcover) | ISBN 9781250780232 (ebook)
Subjects: LCSH: Mental healing. | Self-care, Health. | Mind and body. | Holistic medicine.
Classification: LCC RZ400 .M47 2021 | DDC 615.8/528—dc23
LC record available at https://lccn.loc.gov/2021015927

Our books may be purchased in bulk for promotional, educational, or business use. Please contact your local bookseller or the Macmillan Corporate and Premium Sales Department at 1-800-221-7945, extension 5442, or by email at MacmillanSpecialMarkets@macmillan.com.

First Edition: 2021

10 9 8 7 6 5 4 3 2 1

Dedicated to the memory of
Bernice Donna Mary
(my grandmother "Bee")

Awakening to the Fifth Dimension
has been channeled by
Kimberly's Guides of Christ Light

CONTENTS

FOREWORD

C. Norman Shealy, M.D., Ph.D.,
President of Shealy-Sorin Wellness

In virtually all religions, there is a concept of spiritual healing. Well-known healers such as Oral Roberts and Kathryn Kuhlman kept no written record of their percentage of proven cures. The most studied healer was Olga Worrall, who worked at Mt. Washington United Methodist Church for thirty-six years in Baltimore. She was shown to be able to heal bacteria subjected to antibiotics and make changes in a cloud chamber. I possess fifteen thousand letters she received from grateful patients, but, once again, there is no record of a percent of "cures" she was able to achieve.

I have demonstrated the ability of many healers to raise DHEA, the anti-stress hormone, and especially to change brain EEGs, in two hundred cases, from outside the room, as well as up to one thousand miles away. This is done almost instantly. It suggests that the healer's energy moves at scalar speed, faster than the speed of light.

Kimberly Meredith is an outstanding healer with an

ever-growing number of spectacular healings. I have recorded her altering the EEG of patients from outside the room, apparently focusing scalar energy. This suggests that she taps that mysterious realm of quantum entanglement in a positive way. All empty space in the Universe is filled with scalar energy, and in empty space the size of a helium molecule, there is enough energy to boil the ocean. This energy is the most remarkable evidence of Divine power.

Kimberly has a unique ability to sense areas of the body and mind that need healing and to direct appropriate healing energy to those areas. Other famous healers and intuitives, such as Edgar Cayce, gave a great variety of suggestions for healing, but he did not lay hands on, or focus scalar energy, to the many who consulted him. Caroline Myss is a gifted medical intuitive, but she does not provide spiritual healing.

Kimberly, though still early in her successful spiritual healing work, has the potential to become one of the greatest healers and medical intuitives of this century.

A NOTE TO THE READER

Dear Reader,

This is not your ordinary book on healing. There are many books that can give you advice on how to heal from various diseases, often written by doctors or other health practitioners. Many of those books contain good information.

But this book, while also on healing, is written from a different viewpoint.

As a medical Medium, I have a spiritual worldview. I wrote this book on healing and living in the 5th Dimension from that perspective. Much of this information will be new to you, and I encourage you to read through the book carefully. The advice in this book is powerful, and I hope it will inspire you to explore the 5th Dimension healing in your life.

In addition to spiritual practices that will lift you into the realm of the 5th Dimension, I have included a section that is devoted to practical 5th Dimension healing practices for your mind and body. These are all general recommendations, and I invite you to read through them to find the ones that resonate with you.

You'll see in reading this book that I often work with doctors and other health care professionals, and I feel that healing comes in many forms, through many ways. Working with a health care professional is an important thing to do for all of us. Since every person is unique, and since reading a book is different from having a one-on-one scan from me, this book is not meant to prescribe or diagnose medical treatment. Anytime in discussing our health, it is important to remind the reader to always consult your health practitioner before making changes that could affect your health. Please, do not discontinue or make changes to any medical directive your doctor has given you without consulting your doctor.

Of course, never do any meditative practice while driving or operating machinery of any kind. Above all, use your God-given common sense to always take positive actions.

May this book open a door for you . . . a portal into the 5th Dimension way of thinking and living.

Love yourself and others.

With love,

Kimberly

THE 5D GLOSSARY

Learning the Language of the 5th Dimension

The 5th Dimension (5D) has a different vibration from the 3rd Dimension (3D) world, and therefore it also has a different language. Throughout this book, I use many words and phrases that discuss the 5th Dimension and the spiritual and healing paths. For clarity, I'm including this glossary to help with many of the concepts I discuss. If you find yourself confused while reading the book, refer back to this glossary. Allow the language of the 5th Dimension to uplift and inspire you.

3rd Dimension (3D)—Fear, egotist behavior, greed, dense rules. The 3rd Dimension can be a good or bad reality. The configuration of space with which we are most familiar, comprised of length, width, and height.

4th Dimension (4D)—The connection to astral travel, the higher connections with Angels, your Guides, and animals. The 4th Dimension often brings your soul mate to you. The next higher Dimension above the 3rd Dimension, possessing all three dimensions of length, width, and height, plus an additional Dimension. This is a very important Dimension to say yes and agree with to enter into the 5th Dimension.

5th Dimension (5D)—Pure light, love, linear time lines, and realities. The tapping into your full potential can happen. 5D means you live from your heart and all is possible. The next higher Dimension above the 4th Dimension, possessing two additional dimensions beyond length, width, and height. Existing within this Dimension allows for significantly enhanced Spirituality, consciousness, and emotional and physical health.

12th Dimension (12D)—A process of returning to source. A ray of God Frequency in full physical form. This highly spiritual Dimension possesses nine additional dimensions beyond length, width, and height.

Ascension—The spiritual elevation of an individual, a group, or even an entire world.

Awaken—To become aware of spiritual nature as the primary and fundamental state of being.

Blinking (eye blinks of Kimberly Meredith)—Means of communication with the Spirit World, the Other Side with her many higher-dimensional Guides, and the Holy Spirit.

Chakra—Any of several energetic vortices intersecting individual physical and energetic bodies. Each chakra represents various aspects of an individual's characteristics, as well as physical and emotional well-being.

Channeling—A natural form of communication between humans and Angelic beings, nature spirits, nonphysical entities, or even animals and pets. They allow themselves to sense the nonverbal communication from another being and then translate it into human words. They are hypersensitive humans.

Chanting—A specialized vocal technique. What you chant is often composed for you. Whether you chant, pray, sing, or whisper, you are communicating with God.

Crown Chakra (Sahasrara chakra)—Associated with the pineal gland, little is known about this chakra except that it responds to light. When the cosmic consciousness shines in the mind of humans, humans attain truth.

Dharma—A universal truth and reality term with multiple meanings across multiple religions relating to the eternal nature of reality, cosmic law, the "right way of living," and "path of rightness."

Dark Forces—Groups of souls that have very little light consciousness. When dark forces have power, we give it to them. The opposite is God, the Father, the Divine, the Omnipresent, Spirit, the Universe.

Energy—The form of the entire Universe, including all physical matter; the form that spirits and souls take; the means of conveying positive or negative subtle spiritual influence.

Etheric Angelic Light Language—A unique language spoken by Angels and human channels who receive and convey these Angelic messages.

Feminine Side (not gender)—The female energetic aspect of both females and males. All men and women have a feminine side.

Flow—Best described as a state of consciousness when you feel and perform your best. Within the brain, flow is characterized by four elements: selflessness, timelessness, effortlessness, and richness. Your sense of self vanishes. You're not self-conscious. Your sense of time disappears.

Frequencies—The degree to which spiritual energy is positive or negative.

God Blinks—Kimberly's eyes blink in rapid code. When both eyes blink together at once, this specific code means you had a surgery or a life-threatening event that has been already healed by the Holy Spirit as a Miracle.

God Frequency—It's the direct communication with GOD using your culture language. The human body cellular level that vibrationally connects to heal and feel the Divine presence.

God-Holy Spirit—The Omnipresent energy of the miraculous, gifts of healing, gentle, loving, kind. Our highest conscious choice, a union of love, one with God.

The Guides—Higher-dimensional beings who seek to assist in the uplifting of humanity to reach greater levels of health, Spirituality, and global unity. They communicate in many different ways.

Healing Trilogy—The cooperative energetic confluence between God / the Holy Spirit, a healer, and an individual in need of healing.

Karma—Our day-to-day actions in the 5D reality; it's 100 percent our souls' responsibility.

Law of One—There is only one infinite Creator. We are beings that are one. The Christ Consciousness and the natural laws are governed by our Universe. The RA transmission of light. "I am RA" means the infinite Law of One, the love and light, the infinite Creator.

Light Body—The energetic counterpart of the physical body. When we shift our consciousness from our human bodies to Source and become more connected to the Spirit realm, we can feel and be spiritually and energetically activated.

Masculine Side (not gender)—The male energetic aspect of both males and females. All men and women have a masculine side.

Medical Intuitive—An individual who is able to remotely detect medical conditions within the body of another individual and connect to why the condition occurred without possessing any information about the person.

Medium—An individual who is able to act as a vessel for Spirit Beings, thereby accessing and presenting information from the Spirit Realm, and could be used to describe a "channel." However, the term *Medium* is usually associated with contacting recently departed persons with contact sought by relatives or friends. *Channels*, as we use the term, will usually allow more highly evolved spiritual beings and Spirit teachers to come through and speak. Channels are also capable of doing crossover readings by connecting to and communicating with the spirits of physically deceased humans and animals. Mediums and channels are highly respected because they often have multiple gifts and see ways to help people through their connection with Spirit.

Merkaba—Mer (light) Ka (soul) Ba (body); a sacred, geometric, starlike shape from early Jewish mysticism combining two pyramid shapes, one right side up and one upside down. The word can mean *chariot* or *light spirit body*. The Merkaba can help elevate energy and consciousness.

Miracle—An intervention by the Miraculous Divine and the Spirit Realm on behalf of an individual's well-being.

Mother Mary—The Virgin Mother of Jesus Christ, who is revered worldwide and who acts as an intercessor on behalf of all mankind.

Negative Energy—A low-frequency force or frequency capable of causing harm, illness, discord, and disunity.

Power of Prayer—Communicating powerfully with God. All you have to do is ask God for his help.

Prayer—The power of prayer is the act of speaking through your heart to reach out to the Omnipresent.

Super Consciousness—A super consciousness mind is a level of awareness that sees beyond material reality and taps into the energy of the flow of matter and space and can actually tap into conscious creation.

Shield—An energetic field capable of protecting an individual from harmful negative energy.

Starseed—A person who is spiritually aware, having a strong connection to the Divine Creator. Starseeds are said to have old souls from birth and are sent back to Earth to help with the Ascension. Such persons may display spiritual gifts having all the "clairs" (intuitive abilities). Some Starseeds are able to read minds and have telepathy.

Time—The Dimension the Guides want us to keep moving forward. If time weren't a Dimension, then we would not move forward and we could not construct space-time. We can, however, choose to bounce between time in the higher Dimensions.

Trance State Gate Vortex—A natural hypnotic trance

state that brings out your gifts safely in any place. This can be self-taught.

Trance Channel—A person who is able to set their conscious self aside to allow another being, a nonphysical or Spirit being, to speak through their body. They are able to be in a state of hypnosis, like Edgar Cayce. A trance is the highest form of channeled uttered consciousness. The Guides can help direct great information to support our humanity when they are used correctly.

Zone—A dimensional consciousness where everything is easy and magical and centered on focused dimensional reality without knowing it.

INTRODUCTION

My Journey into the Miraculous

My journey to becoming a medical Medium was unique. Most medical Mediums never have any medical training. In my early teens in Southern California, I started out as a candy striper, which are volunteers at local hospitals. I loved helping out and working in a healing environment. Shortly after, because the staff loved my work, the hospital hired me as an admitting clerk. Not long after, I entered nursing school and got my license as a certified nurse assistant. I worked long hours on many trauma unit floors, and I would float to the units where they needed me most. Meanwhile, I took continuing education courses to become a registered nurse.

I was often sidetracked by the entertainment world. A close friend had sent me to my first hospital television show, called *Strong Medicine*. I was doing what I normally do at the hospital, saying a few words such as, "Give me 5 cc of valium, stat," and "Code blue." I thought this was cool. Then I got an acting agent, and I was totally hooked. I was setting up the IVs on set, setting up all the masks, gowns, and gloves, and I was also often in scenes on camera.

I still worked in the hospital, but after several more jobs, I became known in Hollywood as the go-to expert for on-call nursing and as an on-camera actress and medical adviser. I must have advised over forty films, television shows, and commercials. I was featured in *Emmy* magazine for my work on TV shows such as *Brothers & Sisters*, with Sally Field and Rob Lowe; *All My Children*; *Scrubs*; *General Hospital*; and *The Young and the Restless*. I worked on several seasons of *Grey's Anatomy*, as well as movies like *My Sister's Keeper*, with Cameron Diaz.

My last show was HBO's *Getting On*, where I had just been hired. I was so excited when Laurie Metcalf, the lead actress, came to visit my grandma in the nursing home where she was living at the time. The show was based on a home for elders, and it had a comic English brightness to it. Laurie wanted to see how the senior home was set up and get a feel for the setting. My grandma Bernice was delighted to have a visitor, even though she didn't know who Laurie was. They connected immediately and had a beautiful visit with each other.

At this time in my life, I was ready to take a leave of absence from the hospital to work on the show. For a time, this became my normal—take a leave of absence from the hospital to work on a TV show or film, and then come back when I was finished. I didn't want to leave working in the hospital totally, because I loved helping people in real life.

Working in the hospital, though, started to take its toll. The trauma floor I worked on had felt colder and harder, and many people were passing away at this time. A lot of spiritual paranormal happenings were present on that floor. This was a critical-care unit, and you needed to be tough. I will never forget the smell of death and the sadness. The beautiful actress Elizabeth Taylor and the actor Michael Clarke Duncan of *Green Mile* movie fame passed on that floor while I was working there.

At this time, my hospital supervisor told us that we were short on staff and we would have to take the bodies to the morgue on our own. I looked at my nurse colleague, and she was so upset. The duty of bagging dead bodies was nothing new to me. But going down to the morgue into the cold cement room and pushing this huge bed into a slot was hard work, both physically and emotionally. We knew we were shorthanded, so we had to do what needed to be done.

My life consisted of the Hollywood realities of code blues on set and then the difficult work in the hospital. I felt like I was being pulled in many directions at once. But God had the most unbelievable plan for me I could ever imagine.

Two months later, I ended up as a patient back in the same hospital in which I worked.

Even with my frenetic schedule, I continued visiting my grandmother at the nursing home every other day. There were many people at the nursing home who didn't have family and friends to visit them. It was sad to see people without loved ones to care for them. I wanted to spend time with my grandmother, who always called me "Chon," to make sure she was properly cared for and ensure all was well with her.

When I visited her in the nursing home, I often laid my hands on her to pray, especially when she had difficulty breathing from asthma. I could see how these simple actions would make her breathe easier and bring her peace. I believe that these actions, given freely in love, prolonged her life through the prayers and blessings, and the love and laughter. It's amazing how simple prayer and healing touch can bring more life to others and to ourselves.

MY FIRST NEAR-DEATH EXPERIENCE

Just before Thanksgiving 2012, I was on a sidewalk in Sherman Oaks, California, when an SUV with a broken door hinge had its passenger door fly open, hitting me square in my body and knocking me off my feet. I fell onto the side of the curb, and my head slammed against the concrete surface. My head and jaw hurt, and I was in throbbing pain from this freak accident; but concerned about losing time on my job, I refused to go to a hospital. I fought going to the hospital so hard after I got hit by the car that day. I did everything I could to ignore the pain and stiffness in my neck. I wanted that job more than anything because I was now going to be a full-time medical adviser on the hospital show. I was determined not to let the car accident win, even though day after day, I got dizzier and more dehydrated.

This accident could not have happened at a more inconvenient time. Thanksgiving was around the corner, and after years of hard work, I was finally working in my dream job as a medical consultant on *Getting On*. I was doing what I loved, feeling proud of my professional accomplishments and extremely grateful for the work I was doing. Though after the accident my head hurt and I was in a lot of pain, I decided to tough it out because I didn't want to lose what I had worked so hard to get.

Should I have gone to seek medical advice right then? Probably. But I considered myself tough. I had endured a difficult childhood, I had worked in a trauma center, I had handled many responsibilities and was working constantly. I thought, *I can handle this.* I really believed I could tough it out through the pain, dizziness, and nausea with pain medicine, so I didn't go to the hospital. I took over-the-counter medicine to alleviate the pain, and I went on with my life as if nothing happened.

But I began to vomit and felt sick all over. A few days later, I finally decided to call the doctor, who asked what happened. I told him, "I was hit by a car, and I'm not feeling good. My neck is hurting. It's stiff, and I'm vomiting."

The doctor said, "I think you might have a concussion," and asked me to come into the office to be seen. Instead, I asked him for medicine for the stiffness in my neck.

My boyfriend at the time began to notice something was not right. He said, "You don't look good. Your face is pale, you're vomiting, and you look sick. What did the doctor say?"

I explained that the doctor had prescribed medicine for my neck. "My neck is just a little stiff, but I'm okay. I'm still doing the show."

He was concerned. "Kimberly, you don't look good."

In hindsight, I should have stopped everything and taken care of this, but I wasn't thinking clearly. The entire time, I was telling myself, *There's no way I'm going to give up the life I've worked so hard for. I've got my own show now, and I'm going on with the show.*

By now, it was the third week of November, and even though I was in severe pain, I arrived at work for the show.

My head throbbed and felt like it would explode. I was on set doing medical consulting while continuing to take more and more pain relief medication, trying to cope. The director had no idea what happened to me, because of course I didn't tell anyone. He continued to ask work-related questions. "Kimberly, where should we set up the shot? Where should we do the lines?" Still my head was pounding, and intense chills were going through my body. I finally started to admit that something wasn't right. During lunch, everyone was eating, but I had to go lie down in my car. The injury was progressing.

Thanksgiving arrived, and during dinner, I lay down in the bedroom because my head still hurt. I heard, "Where's Kimmie?" My boyfriend came into the bedroom to check on me. "I'm really sick!" I exclaimed.

He was adamant. "You have *got* to go to the doctor."

Instead of going to the doctor, I just called in to the doctor's office for another prescription. This time, the doctor refused and said, "We're not going to give you any more medicine. You've got to come in."

I refused. I told him, "No, I've got to finish this season of the TV show." By then, I was getting worse. My bladder hurt, and I was having difficulty urinating. My head was constantly throbbing. By the time we wrapped the show, I was barely walking.

Looking back, I wish I had taken medical action earlier, but again, I was trying to keep the job that I loved and stay tough through it all. When I look back at this time, the irony of my being in the medical field and refusing medical help is not lost on me. I was being stubborn, trying to hold everything together, afraid that my absence would jeopardize my dream job. Believe me, I don't advise others to be as stubborn as I was.

One month later, on Christmas Eve, I got up out of bed and collapsed. I fell onto the floor and started to vomit. My boyfriend found me on the floor. He took me to Cedars-Sinai Medical Center. The situation had gotten so bad that the doctors told my boyfriend, "Her kidneys are shutting down. We have to take her into ICU. She needs an MRI. What happened with her?"

That evening, a nurse injected me with blood thinners, and my blood pressure began to drop. I actually saw it drop down to zero, and that was when I blacked out. All of a sudden, everything became blurry, then I saw an image of me alone on the other side, that fine line between life here and life after death. During the time I blacked out, I was not afraid.

While passing into that other side, I first experienced an indescribable white light and soft circles that were floating around me. Then I heard the sounds of the nurses' voices, which began to fade out. I went through a tunnel and saw the beautiful white light and also misty soft clouds. I walked through white clouds, and there were tiny white lights everywhere. While I stood in the white light, there were soft, blurred images of faces. There were purple roses everywhere, and I felt the strong presence and connection with my ancestors, including my Italian shaman grandmother. I felt the energy of our Creator around me, holding me. I could hear soft whispers say to me, "You're okay. Everything is okay," while at the same time, I heard the faint voices of the nurses. It was comforting, beautiful, and peaceful. I knew something was going on. I had left my body. I saw myself outside my body while I experienced another Dimension of myself. I had been lifted by the Holy Spirit. I had been graced by the Angels and God, to the other side, and then I surrendered. Then, I awakened with a gasp of air and had absolutely no fear of death.

Soon after, I felt a deep pressure, like a ball on my chest, and a blinding bright light through my eyes. I heard a demanding voice say, "You're going to eat!" I gasped for air again, and a huge white ball of light pounded down onto me again with amazing energy on my chest. This energy wouldn't lift up, and I was bound to the bed with it pressing down on me. I wasn't aware of what was going on at this time, and I was frightened. I asked God to get off me.

I was given an order: "You are chosen to heal cancer and diseases."

My breath came back into my body, and then calmness came over me, and I felt better. When I tried to wake up, there was only white light.

When I returned to my body and woke up, the doctors were pulling and poking me. I was very confused. I didn't know what had happened. I was very sick and felt chills all over my neck and body. I also couldn't move my legs without trembling. I felt an amazing number of chills going through my legs. I truly believe the trembling was the Holy Ghost appearing through my body, helping me to witness that the Christself within had risen. God had brought me back, and now I was tasked with accepting the light and Awakening to my gifts.

After the near-death experience (NDE), I underwent test after test after test. I had intravenous (IV) units attached to me and probes attached to my head. I couldn't feel my legs, and I couldn't walk. I then started to lose my speech. I didn't talk or sound the way I do now prior to the accident. My pronunciation was completely different. I had a totally different sound to my voice. With all of this going on, I stayed in the hospital for almost three months. I couldn't believe what was happening to me.

During the months of hospital stay, I frequently called my grandmother at the nursing home where she was being cared for. She pleaded with me, "Can you get me out of here? I need to see you."

I felt terrible because her health had declined while I was in the hospital and I wasn't physically able to visit her. When we talked on the phone, she offered me encouragement, demanding of me, "Pull yourself up by your bootstraps. Get up out of there and come see me."

Nurses were coming into my room at 4:00 every morning and giving me heparin shots, which bruised my stomach and left me weak, dizzy, and constipated. The nurses were kind, and I knew some of them because I had worked there. I was having daily prayers with both a rabbi and a priest and had a spiritual counselor teaching me transcendental meditation, which I had never heard of before. My physical therapy moved slowly, and I couldn't take five steps from my bed, even after one month. I was losing hope. I saw several neurologists, and they decided to put me in a wheelchair and continue my rehab.

During my rehab, I started to listen to my headset, getting inspiration from listening to rap music, including "Lose Yourself" by Marshall Mathers (Eminem) over and over again. Something about that song helped me to gain strength and healing. Even after I went home, I continued listening to his music as part of my therapy.

One day, a physical therapist took me downstairs in my wheelchair to get something to drink. Unbeknownst to me, the producer from the show I worked on had the flu and was at the hospital pharmacy to pick up his prescription. I couldn't believe that of all the pharmacies in LA, he was here in this one! I didn't want anyone to see me like this, or even to know I was sick, let alone see me in a wheelchair, but of course, he noticed me. "Kimberly," he asked with great concern, "what are you doing in a wheelchair?" I was so embarrassed and worried about not being able to work and didn't know what to say. Sure enough, after seeing the producer, I got a call from someone at the show inquiring, "Kimberly, are you going to be able to come back to work? What's going on with you?"

I told them I had an accident and I wasn't sure what was going to happen with my health. But I knew in my heart that sadly, I would have to give up my job because I could no longer walk.

"I'm never going to be the same," I said to the nurse wheeling me back to my room.

At first, my boyfriend came to visit me every day he could get off work, and then his visits tapered off. Everything I wanted, everything I worked so hard for, was gone. I spent many nights by myself in the stillness of the hospital room reflecting and crying, but I continued to pray to God to stop the pain.

In addition to being afraid that I was going to lose my job,

I felt extremely guilty that I wasn't able to be at the nursing home to help my grandmother. When I finally did get out of the hospital, I still couldn't get over to the nursing home, because I was in a wheelchair. It was a very sad and difficult time for me.

One of the last times I saw my grandmother, I was in the wheelchair. She wasn't breathing very well, but she said, "Chon, you're here." She was so happy to see me.

Five days later, when my grandmother passed, the nursing home attendant called me an hour before to say she wasn't doing well. Still needing assistance to walk, I couldn't get myself out of bed, so I couldn't get to the nursing home to watch my grandmother pass and witness her last breath. It was devastating for me to not be with her.

My grandmother Bernice died at ninety-five years old, three months after my car accident. This completely changed my life. My grandmother was my soul mate. I believe we lived many lives together and that this is why I always wanted to be with her. She passed and we were once again separated, but now she's with me from the other side. I know she wants me back with her, and I know we will be together again. We have reincarnated in many lives together, and it will happen again.

I think of her often and remember her special knock, a particular old-fashioned knock that was used during the vaudeville era known as "Shave and a Haircut, Two Bits," a seven-note musical call-and-response. She used it in a light-hearted and playful manner with family and friends, to announce her arrival. She would knock on her glass when she wanted something. Even though she is gone, I can sometimes still hear that knock. She was my constant source of emotional support, safety, and unconditional love during times when I felt alone and misunderstood. Our connection was strong and eternal on many levels. The realm between my grandmother in my life before and now is completely different. That will make a big difference in the future because there is a big difference in me now, as I've walked into a different Dimension.

A year and a half after my grandmother died, I began blinking frequently, which I would come to realize was my way of connecting to Spirit after the NDE. It reminded me of when I was with her as a child, I sometimes blinked in rapid patterns, and I didn't always know why I blinked in such unusual ways or what, if anything, the blinking meant. But she somehow knew it was okay for me and would encourage it, and I knew it was good. Eventually, growing up, I stopped blinking in that unusual way. But now, after she passed, this fluttering of my eyelids returned. It was then that I understood that after my NDE in the hospital and after my beloved grandmother passed, this was when my mediumship awakened. Further, I learned that it was my God-gifted form of blinking that was to be the method of communication between me and the Divine. I'll share more about my unique form of blinking, from my childhood to its reappearance.

BROUGHT BACK INTO THE LIGHT

My next near-death experience happened several weeks later, after I returned home from the hospital. By then, I was up and able to walk around, though I also still used the wheelchair often. I weighed 105 pounds and was not doing well. I was still experiencing the effects of the concussion and remained weak. Rocky, my eighty-pound American bulldog, however, still needed to be walked. I remember the day was overcast and dreary. There was a gardener with a leaf blower outside close to my home while I slowly walked Rocky. As the gardener approached us, his very loud leaf blower caused Rocky to become alarmed. Not wanting to make Rocky more upset, I asked the gardener to please move aside to let us by. He looked at me with anger and pushed the leaf blower into Rocky's face. Rocky barked and lunged at him, which threw me into the center of the street.

I landed on my head and blacked out and began seeing and hearing Angels, skeletons, and many faces all around me. I felt the cold of the hard pavement and warm blood on the back of my head. I felt myself floating above the street, being supported by the Angels and looking down at Rocky. I whispered, "Help me, please. Someone help me!" But no one could hear me.

Like an Angel, Rocky never left my side. I felt his licks on my face while I lay on the pavement. I went in and out of seeing things from both perspectives, from my worldly surroundings and from the other side. Amazingly, not one car hit me, even though I was lying in the middle of the street, because Rocky stood upright and shielded me like a guardian Angel. I truly believe my dog was my protective Angel. I was experiencing hazy faces of onlookers from the street, mixed with darker spirits coming in and out from the other side. Yet the Angels were also holding me up as these darker spirits appeared to me like skeletons.

I finally woke up after seeing those extremes of light and dark from the other side. I knew I had experienced another Miracle. I saw the entirety of the dark side trying to come to me, but I was saved by the love of the Angels. I awoke to see my dog with me in the middle of the street and many people gathered around me.

There was blood on the back of my head, and I was experiencing a tremendous amount of pain in the same area where I had the previous concussion. It was a Miracle I lived again and that my dog never left my side—I had survived another NDE.

Since these NDEs, the last four years of my life have been completely different from the life I once knew. Everything about my life drastically changed. I don't feel, look, walk, or talk the same as I did prior to the NDEs. I know my NDEs are still being experienced within me.

We all live in a multidimensional world, and God heals us through His grace and time. Following this second NDE, I was upstairs in my bedroom a lot and couldn't walk down the stairs without assistance, I felt depressed and cried all the time. Yet I could sense the presence of Mother Mary coming to me. I saw a vision of her staring down at me while surrounded by the holy water of Lourdes, the healing site in France. When I was asleep, I kept dreaming of her. I didn't know what I was going to do with myself. I prayed to God and repeatedly asked, "What is the plan here? What's happening? What's going to happen to me?"

THE BEGINNINGS OF MEDIUMSHIP AND HEALING GIFTS

A friend I used to attend Mass with, Sarah, a nurse and a Reiki practitioner, came to see me about three weeks after I got out of the hospital. We used to do medical consulting work together. She was heartbroken when I lost the job on the HBO medical series *Getting On*, because she knew how hard it was to get a break onto a show. She came over after work one day and found me on my knees crying. I was still in so much pain. The medicine the doctors had prescribed was not working.

She said, "Look at me! I'm going to lay my hands on your head, and we're going to pray. I'm going to help to take this pain out of your head at last."

I said, "Yes, please help me! This medicine is not working. I'm in so much pain."

She kept her hands on my head and prayed out loud, declaring my healing. She kept praying, but it didn't seem to work very well.

After she left, I continued to pray to be healed. I prayed and prayed and prayed. I wanted a solution, and I decided I had to do something differently from before. I grabbed the gigantic bag of medicine I had and threw the pills all down the toilet. I vowed, "God, I'm not going to take another pill for the rest of my life." And that was it, even to this day. I decided to take the Divine guidance within me and lay my hands on my head and pray. I did this every day until the pain left. Prayer is a positive way to connect with the high vibrational energy that resonates with our breath. I also started saying the Hail Mary prayer. You might be familiar with it:

Hail Mary, full of grace,
The Lord is with thee.
Blessed art thou among women,
and blessed is the fruit of thy womb, Jesus.
Holy Mary, Mother of God,
pray for us sinners, now,
and at the hour of our death. Amen.

Something started to spark from the Hail Mary practice along with my laying my own hands on myself. I was being healed. It's somehow divinely appropriate that I was the first person I laid my hands on. They were teaching me to heal myself.

During the night, I began to channel the Hail Marys. Channeling was a form of communication and education, happening on a different Dimension within. I didn't know anything about how to channel, but it was happening through me. My Spirit Guides, all holy and higher Angelic beings, would wake me up with the channeling during the night, asking me to trust what they were telling me to tell the Universe. During the night, I began to wake up reciting the Hail Mary prayer. What I came to learn was that I was beginning to channel a higher wisdom, which I came to know as *the Guides*. They would wake me up at night and give me messages about life. They were teaching me about what I came to know was the 5th Dimension, and their wisdom was outstanding. I soaked up everything they taught me. They were healing my body in the 5th Dimension and Awakening the gifts I had been born with.

If someone had seen me, they might have thought it was odd, but all these experiences were not only soothing, they were inspiring me. I was hungry for more. There would be times when I woke with my arms flapping like Angel wings or my arms formed into the triangle of the Holy Trinity symbol, or my body moved to form the shape of a cross. Also, at that time, while asleep at night, my Angels would come to me to give me messages and form my hands in the sign of the Trinity. The Trinity is a triangular symbol meaning you, me, and the Holy Spirit. The Holy Spirit is the center of the Trinity, which holds us all together. This might have seemed strange for a girl who was raised Jewish, having been born in Lynwood, California, to an Italian Catholic mother who converted to Judaism. The Guides, though, clearly have no religion, and they wanted me to embody the essence of Mother Mary. I often see Mother Mary and Jesus, who represent the Divine love here for us all, when I am doing my healing work.

Waking up in the middle of the night became commonplace for me. In addition to my Angels, I also was astounded to have the Spirit of Albert Einstein wake me at night. The Angels and Albert would stand over me and teach me about dimensional theory, how to move humanity into Christ Consciousness, and how to remain in this consciousness.

Not everything that I was experiencing came from the Angels, Mother Mary, the Guides, or Albert Einstein. One night, early on, when I finally accepted my gifts, I awoke with a flash of red light in my face, a pressure on my throat, and my necklace with a cross pendant taken off my neck. It felt stifling and uncomfortable. I got out of bed and walked downstairs to get some water and was surprised to find my cross pendant and necklace on the floor beside the fireplace where I would do my healing. When I found the cross pendant on the floor, it felt like I was being warned to not do God's work.

During that entire week, I had many signs of dark energies that came to me with warnings not to proceed with the healing work. It was at this time that I made a spiritual, emotional, and mental declaration that I would have faith in God's healing energy. I made it loud and clear to the dark energy that I am not in fear, and I made a full commitment to my calling.

Three months later, as I continued to pray on myself, a family member sent me what's called a cold laser machine to help heal my neck. My girlfriend came over, and thankfully, she knew how to use it and helped me give myself my first treatment.

The cold laser machine is something that has been around for years. According to what I learned, most people would need to do twenty-four to sixty treatments to heal most physical ailments. In my case, I was told that I would need hundreds of treatments for my neck and my brain to fully heal. My friend taught me how to use the machine on myself, and so I began. To my surprise, I saw improvements after three or four treatments. This was miraculous. It was God.

The more I worked with the cold laser machine and the more my gifts were emerging, the more I felt a connection to the spiritual energies of Albert Einstein and now also with Edgar Cayce, known as the Sleeping Prophet. I didn't know who Cayce was until people began commenting that my mediumship resembled Cayce's, who entered a trance when he channeled about people's health challenges. That's true for me, too.

What is important to know is that before it was possible for any healing to occur, I first had to have the understanding and belief that I could be healed. With that understanding, I began to heal myself with God through the laser machine. The light from the laser machine worked as a conduit of God, and I was able to continue my self-healing. In the midst of excruciating pain, and knowing that the life I had known before these events was forever gone, I relied on my decision to trust in God. I put 100 percent of my faith in God and not in the dark energy that I felt was whispering to me in my mind that I would not be able to make it and that I would live in a wheelchair for the rest of my life with a brace around my neck.

As a result of my healing process, I began to consider a larger possibility. *If it worked on me,* I thought, *it can work on others.* I knew I couldn't go back to my old life. So I made the decision to stop trying to control so much in my life, and instead let go and flow with whatever was going to happen. It was from that point that everything started to unfold organically through God. The doctors saw my healing progression and were astounded by the visible improvements. I told them it was from prayer with my hands and the cold laser machine.

Inspired by my progress, I decided to get training and

become licensed to perform cold laser therapy. I found a place to take a class in Marina del Rey. I was still in pain while taking the class, but I kept doing the laser, learning more about how to do it and how to regenerate tissue. I was ahead of the other people in the class because I knew so much about the machine already from my practice of it on myself.

One day a friend, who was an agent in Los Angeles, came to my home and asked if I could pray on his injured Achilles tendon and help him. I rubbed my hands together and prayed and said the Hail Mary while placing my hands on his Achilles tendon. I grabbed the cold laser handle and punched a few numbers on the machine and put it on his Achilles tendon for about two seconds. He said thank you and went home.

Two days later, he called me and said, "Kimberly, they canceled my surgery and did an X-ray, and my Achilles is completely healed. You are a healer!"

Up to that point, I had never thought of myself as a healer. I didn't even know what being a healer meant.

He shared his success story at Gold's Gym in Venice Beach, California, telling people I had healed him with my prayers and the cold laser and that the cold laser and I were a conduit to God. The word of my healing ability spread like wildfire.

Soon after, I had athletes coming to my house for treatments. I laid my hands on them and did my prayers and used the cold laser. A professional boxer with a rotator cuff tear came to visit me and asked me to try the laser on him. I went across his shoulders with my hands and correctly diagnosed the problem area. He said, "I've been in pain for months. What are you going to do?"

I said, "I'm going to pray on you, and you can pray with me. Let's heal it."

I prayed on him, and all the swelling went down. I only did a little bit of the laser. He commented how my hands felt hot and had a healing effect on him. He said, "I'm so grateful. I will spread your name all around the gym and send more people to you. But first, I think you should get a better table for people to lie on. This one is not strong enough." I thought, *I'm not doing much right now, and there will be no more TV or movie consulting or working at the hospital. I felt that God had taken me out of that world. What am I going to do? How am I going to live here?* So I said, "I'm in," and he started to send people to me.

The cold laser ended up healing the boxer fully in only two sessions, which shocked his doctor. The boxer was also a trainer at Gold's Gym, and he sent me even more clients. They would lie down, and I used my hands to find out where the problem was coming from. I would take out the energy that blocked the flow of blood in the veins, and they would breathe it out. Some would come and just ask that I pray with them. They were getting a lot of relief, and this got me even more recognition.

In addition to what I was already doing, I started to rub my hands together and call in the 5th Dimensional energy, that realm of miracles where your consciousness is opened to your heart frequency. As I rubbed my hands together and prayed, I would touch the clients while they also prayed, and the stronger they prayed, the more their joints and ligaments moved back into place and their emotional and physical injuries were healed.

I now know that my two NDEs were destined to happen. Those experiences, while painful, awakened my healing ability and changed the course of my life. I am truly grateful for the healing gifts that were bestowed on me.

Not long after getting my laser license and as my gifts were emerging, my friend Sarah took me to a Reiki class, where I felt my hands getting hotter and hotter as I practiced the techniques on other people. I got my Reiki master license quickly.

My Reiki teacher was impressed by my progress and asked me, "What do you see around people?" I answered that I can see souls and colors. I see tiny sparkling lights around people and in people. She then told me, "You are a full Medium, and I think you will develop your own kind of teachings one day."

She sent me to a famous shaman in Malibu, so she, too, could evaluate my gifts. I felt very honored to be there. She did a drumming ceremony on me, during which I passed out for an hour.

The shaman looked at my hands and told me, "You are channeling the Holy Spirit and many Ascended Masters." I asked her if I could study with her, and she said no. "You are our teacher!"

THE REAPPEARANCE OF THE BLINKING

My grandmother encouraged my unique way of blinking (when I say, "My blinking," you'll know I mean this unique way of fluttering my eyes). Here's what happened. As early as six months old, my parents and other relatives began to notice that I frequently blinked. They thought it was fascinating, but it began to annoy my mother. My paternal grandfather actually followed me around with an 8 mm camera, recording my blinking as I lay in my crib, looking up at everyone, and when I began to crawl around and explore my surroundings.

Being a curious child periodically got me into trouble. While crawling around the house, I found some highly toxic drain cleaner when my uncle was supposed to be watching me. I pulled the bottle down, and the Drano spilled all over my body, causing severe skin burns. When my uncle found me, he put me into the bathtub, flushed water all over me. He also noticed I had swallowed some and rushed me to the hospital to have my stomach pumped. Considering the amount of Drano I consumed and the amount that covered my body, doctors expressed amazement that I had survived.

When I was two years old, growing up in Southern California, my father, Kendall, whom I adored, was drafted into the Vietnam War and sent overseas. The resulting long separation from my father eventually took a toll on my mother, and she filed for divorce. My father didn't learn of the divorce until he returned from Vietnam and then he discovered that my mother had already married another man.

Consistently left hungry and unattended to by my mother, who had developed a drinking problem, I once climbed up onto the bathroom sink to get the baby aspirin, which I thought was candy. I opened the bottle and ate almost half of it. My mother found me unconscious on the floor and drove me to the hospital, where my stomach had to be pumped again.

A family friend who had just returned from Vietnam with my father mentioned how I was such a pretty baby and gifted me with an unusual Vietnamese name, Chon. All the family and friends called me Chon. For many years, I believed Chon meant "pretty baby." Years later, my Reiki master told me Chon meant "God" in Vietnamese. In English, it means "to appoint" or "to choose." Grandmother Bernice had been unknowingly calling me God all of those years.

In contrast to the chaos I felt around my mother, I had an extreme yearning for the loving energy of Bernice Donna Mary Wink, my German paternal grandmother. She was beautiful, with thick black hair, and I felt a tremendous sense of ease and comfort just looking at her. She was the rock of our family. More than anything, I remember feeling my grandmother's soul. I couldn't articulate it, but even at such a young age, I recognized my connection to her soul.

In kindergarten, the other kids noticed that I had unusual palms, filled with a lot of lines, and they refused to hold my hands. When I was born, my father did mention to my grandmother there were unusual lines present on the palms of my hands and soles of my feet. He also told my grandmother when I was born how he felt an indescribable love for me. When he visited me in the nursery as a newborn, he saw the glow of a yellow light around me. It was the happiest day of his life.

For years, I would ask my grandmother about my hands, if they looked strange, or if something was wrong with them. She would say, "No, they're fine. They're good."

When I was four years old, I was outside with my paternal grandfather, Lloyd, at his home in Long Beach, California, learning how to ride a bicycle, when I found a dead bird. I'm not sure why I decided to do this, but it felt instinctual. I laid my hands on the bird and began to pray over it. To my surprise, the bird miraculously began to move around in an effort to flap its wings. It had come back to life! I didn't know what to think. I tried to ignore it and tell myself that it did not really happen, but that didn't last for very long. I finally went inside to tell my grandmother about it. She came outside to see the bird and seemed surprised but then made a comment about my maternal great-grandmother Josephina, who was known in the family as a healer herself: "Maybe you're taking after her with healing abilities."

Beside my grandmother's house stood a grapefruit tree. She and I often sat underneath the tree on a swing as she read to me. While I sat on her lap, I often heard a whisper in my right ear, "You're special. You're special. You're special."

"Did you say I was special?" I would ask my grandmother.

"No, I haven't said anything," she would reply.

Throughout my childhood, I repeatedly heard a whisper in my right ear while I sat on my grandmother's lap. I now believe it was Spirit whispering in my ear. I also constantly put my hands on her throat and said, "Swallow, Grandma."

She would tell me, "That's my Adam's apple."

I continued, saying, "I need to put my fingers in there to heal you." I later found out my grandmother suffered from asthma.

As soon as I could write on my own, I wrote little notes to my grandmother that read, "Grandma, don't ever die." I left them around the house for her to find. She would find them and say, using a nickname she had for me, "Kimmie Chon, there's a time to live and a time to die."

I replied to her, "When I speak to God, Grandma, I'll make a new arrangement."

My grandmother took me to see *The Sound of Music,* which was playing in the nearby movie theater. My mother, who was secretly jealous of my relationship with my grandmother, insisted on coming with us. My grandmother, who always dressed immaculately in linen, dressed me in a plaid dress, while my mother wore a sexy Italian dress. During the movie, my mother left the theater and was gone for quite a while. All of a sudden, we heard a loud scream in the movie theater. My mother, in very high heels, had tripped and fell on the ramp while flirting with one of the movie attendants and sprained her ankle. I loved the movie and felt sad when my grandmother took my hand and said, "We have to leave, Kimmie Chon."

Later, my mother felt bad about the incident and having to leave the movie early, so she took me to another movie. She had been drinking, and when we arrived at the theater box office, she looked up at the marquee and saw it was an adult theater, but still purchased tickets for us. The box office attendant did not see me standing beside her, below the counter. When we entered the theater, it was very dark, but we could see men doing inappropriate things in the theater. The film was clearly an adult pornographic film. Her intentions were good, but once again, her naivete and poor judgment caused me to see a dark side of life I should never have seen.

The Sound of Music movie and the convent where the nuns gathered and prayed in the film had made a big impression on me. Although I was too young to know exactly why, something in the film resonated deeply within me, and I began to pray a lot. I asked my grandmother, "What is a nun?"

"Someone who devotes their life to the Lord," she explained.

"What is the Lord?" I asked her.

"It is God."

"What is God?"

She replied, "God is an energy that takes care of you."

I didn't really understand what that was, but even at this young age, I knew in my body it was something greater than all of us. I felt at peace knowing I was taken care of by this energy. I knew the difference in the energy I felt around this woman, my beloved grandmother, whose disposition was honest, sweet, kind, and gentle—the energy of God. In my eyes, she was beauty personified.

The words—*sister* and *nun*—came to me at an age when I didn't understand the significance, but I was so infatuated with being a nun that I wore a nun's white scarf, like a nun's habit, on my head up until the age of nine. Many years later, it now makes sense to me. I believe that in a previous life, I was a sister, that I reincarnated from a convent after having served many lives as a nun.

Though we were Jewish and went to temple on Fridays, we also celebrated Christmas at our home. As I got older, I often walked to Catholic church by myself, and I loved feeling the energy of Jesus and angels around me. Throughout all the extreme difficulties I was experiencing at home, praying to God was a constant source of relief that helped me endure and survive the abuse.

As a child, it was difficult for me to face the dark energy

from the mistreatment by my mother. My father became more and more suspicious that I was being emotionally and physically abused. He went to court in an attempt to get full custody of me, but he failed because back then mothers were given preferential treatment by the court.

I often slept with a small Bible, my great-grandmother's Bible, that had Mother Mary on the cover, and it gave me a lot of strength. Amid the turmoil, I talked to God constantly and felt the presence around me during my dreams and upon awakening early in the morning.

Once in elementary school, we were instructed to line up in pairs and hold hands with a classmate. The little boy who stood in line beside me said he didn't want to hold my hand, complaining there were too many lines on my hands and they felt rough, like something was wrong with both me and my hands. I said that my hands had been reincarnated and God forgot to change my hands. He later told the principal I had said, "My hands are reincarnated."

That afternoon, my mother received a call from the school to come into the principal's office for a meeting. She arrived at the school, and during the meeting, the principal asked her, "Why is she talking about being reincarnated?"

My mother was angry and embarrassed. "I've never told her about reincarnation. I don't know what she's talking about."

After the meeting, we left the principal's office and walked to the car. Before I could reach for the car door handle, I was slapped across the face for using the word *reincarnated* and told to never, ever say that word again.

Throughout my life, I've been drawn to churches and temples and always felt open to learning about various religions and their saints. Although I feel I was born with innate gifts, they were pushed down by my upbringing, then after the NDEs, they emerged again, clearly in full activation now.

As I described earlier, my mother didn't know why I repeatedly blinked for no apparent reason. She knew something was special about me, that I had special abilities, because she witnessed several paranormal events that made her uncomfortable. But when I blinked like that as a child, my mother often would yell at me to stop. We have these gifts from God when we come into the world, as I now know, and sometimes dark energy moves through people, like our parents or a primary caregiver, and the true identity of who we are is pushed away or suppressed.

Once, when my mother, stepfather, and I were in their bedroom, they sat me down on their bed, and I could not stop blinking.

"Why are you blinking like that?" my mother demanded.

I stuttered, "I don't know."

She continued to nervously insist, "Stop blinking!"

While blinking, I felt an energy coming through, and I sensed that I was receiving information. I just didn't yet know what it was. But I also saw how frightened both my mother and stepfather were by the blinking, and because of their fear, I stopped. From that point, at the age of seven on, through determined mental effort, I forced myself to stop the blinking.

After that day, I felt an enormous amount of sadness and depression, feeling like I had lost a deep connection or even my best friend. While I made my mother happy by no longer blinking, and I wanted my mother to be happy because I loved her, despite her abuse and struggles with alcohol dependence, it felt like I had sacrificed an important part of me. That part of me would not be rediscovered until well into adulthood.

My mother, unfortunately, passed away at an early age from substance abuse and depression, even though she had been sober for eight years before relapsing. Despite the abuse I experienced from her, I loved and forgave her.

ANOTHER HEALING GIFT FROM GOD

In May 2015, as I was driving to a client's house, out of nowhere, I started to spontaneously blink again. Two days prior to this, I experienced an Awakening with God. A large ray of light energy came to me while I was sitting on my couch, and I was blinded by the white light passing over my eyes. The significance of this is that my eyes awakened and were blinking again for the first time since I was seven years old.

This was another healing gift from God as a result of the NDE. The blinking began communicating at a higher vibrational code. The only way I can describe it is to say it looks like an eye coming in and out of the light. I often have this in the mornings now; I see an eye coming in and out. It's beautiful. It's the Divine coming to me and speaking to me. When the blinking began, the eye continued to come in and out, which made it difficult for me to see.

With the channeling ability coming out stronger in me, my sight and hearing now became more sensitive. When I worked on clients, I started to ask them if I could use them as a sample to ask yes-or-no questions. The energy of the Divine was speaking to me through my eyes, and I would ask yes-or-no questions to see if I was correct about what medical conditions I found as I interpreted what the energy revealed. For many months, I only asked yes-or-no questions when I scanned the body with my eyes. The Guides taught me how to telepathically blink in these codes. I spoke to Spirit with questions, and they blinked back the answers. Then one night, I had a dream.

In the dream, God assisted me with the healing and said, "We want you to take it [negative energy] out of people and heal them."

I could now blink while in a hypnotic state and find everything unhealthy in a person's body through blinking and scanning them with my hands! I began doing this faster and faster, and then it was transforming into me using both my eyes and hands in psychic surgery, through connection with the Divine.

The significance of the instructions I receive from my Guides through my blinking is as follows:

When my right eye blinks, it is negative energy.

When my left eye blinks, it is positive energy.

When both eyes blink, the negative energy has been successfully transmuted with God and is gone.

My gifts manifest through my eyes, blinking dozens of multidimensional codes. I communicate through Divinely guided sign language, and I also speak in 5th Dimensional Etheric Angelic Light Language (a unique language spoken by Angels and human channels) in order to heal, awaken, and move humanity forward.

What needs to be clear is that with all problems in the

body, the only way negative energy (fear) can attach and manifest through you is if you don't have love fully integrated within you. If you are truly in faith and alignment with the Divine, there is no room for negative energy to reside in your body. This is the fundamental reason why it is imperative that you are 100 percent in dedicated faith with God. People who are fully in faith with God, which is love, can be healed because being in the 5th Dimension connects you to God, making all healing possible.

HOW TO ENTER THE 5TH DIMENSION
Crystals and Meditation

Entering the 5th Dimension requires a different type of awareness, one that notices the synchronicities in life. (Synchronicities are meaningful patterns of what we call coincidences.) Instead of seeing events as co-incidences, we realize they are spiritual guidance. By realizing that things aren't just happenstance and that everything happens for a reason, we enter a higher state of consciousness.

You'll read about a number of ways to enter this higher state. **Crystals** are one way to help us achieve a 5th Dimension mindset. They are like spiritual magnifying glasses, amplifying the power of Spirit in our lives. For instance, amethyst is a stone that helps us to see with more clarity. It stimulates the third eye, giving us a deeper insight into what is really happening in our lives. This provides an invaluable state of awareness that helps us ascend to enter the 5th Dimension if you aren't setting aside time to tune inward and calm the chaos in your mind.

Meditation is the door that leads us into the higher dimensions, yet so many people struggle to sit quietly for any amount of time. Don't make meditation so difficult. Just breathe and focus. Do so for at least five minutes a day. You can meditate in any number of ways, whatever feels right for you. For example, you can put your favorite music on and make the music your meditation. You can take a walk and connect to whatever nature is around you. Or you can sit in a quiet place, breathe deeply, and concentrate on the word *love* or *peace* or *God.* (Just remember not to try to meditate while driving or operating machinery of any kind, or doing anything that requires your attention.)

While you can meditate without them, crystals can help us in our meditation. I find the metaphysical properties of amethyst make it the best crystal for meditation. This crystal can aid in quieting the mind to help us get into a meditative state, connect with the higher self, and assist with the self-discovery process, helping to bring deeper understanding.

Crystals not only connect to all of our chakras, but they also balance our emotional connection to the human and Spirit world. This takes us into the 5th Dimension. The ultimate stones are rose quartz, celestite, amethyst, topaz, and selenite.

Add crystals when you meditate, which is very

healing, but don't wait to have crystals to begin meditating. Begin meditating now, even for a couple minutes at a time. Don't struggle, don't judge yourself, and don't worry that you are doing it wrong. Start where you are.

We have free will and the right to make a choice to be with God or not, to build intimacy and a close relationship. God is an Omnipresent loving energy, and we all have the capability as humans to accept and live in that energy. I honor the Holy Spirit (God energy). By truly accepting the Holy Spirit, we are one with God, and with this connection, healing is possible because we are multidimensional beings and God is a higher frequency. Once you have witnessed a healing Miracle and experienced this higher Dimension, it is easier to reenter that 5th Dimension and beyond.

Even people who don't believe in God, who don't accept the presence of the Holy Spirit, can shift and experience healing once they have witnessed the demonstrations of miraculous healings in others by the Holy Divine. They get awakened by being witnesses and by being in the presence of the miraculous.

The first time I realized my bare hands could dissolve a solid mass tumor was also in 2015. A woman had come to me with a breast lump. As we prayed together in my apartment, chanting the Hail Mary in unison, her breast lump suddenly and completely vanished.

Afterward, we sat together and cried. I stared at my hands

and felt chills running through my body. I felt joy, shock, and, above all, gratefulness. I thought, *WOW! This is it! This is what I am supposed to do! This is real!*

I had flashbacks to my childhood experiences of healing animals. But those events were not like this. I felt deep sensations of astral travel and trance channeling. It was so surreal.

This is not me, I thought. *This is the miraculous using me. We both tapped into that frequency of God and did this! And now the tumor is gone! This is totally cool!*

I wondered if I would teach this in the future. I felt my Guides reply, "Yes."

Since my near-death experiences, the reappearance of my blinking, and the initiation of my medical mediumship and healing work, the last seven years of my life have been completely different from the life I once knew. I don't feel, look, walk, or talk the same as I did prior to the NDEs. In many ways, my near-death experiences are still being experienced.

I wouldn't trade this experience today for anything, because I now feel this is truly who I am and truly who I was meant to be. I am here to serve humanity, and I love what I am blessed to do.

It's true that our world is challenged by a dark energy, and it always has been. I could see this energy before the NDEs, but even more so after those experiences. Now I can see the worst in people and the brightest in them. It is much clearer and more apparent now.

It's as if I am being used like a telephone pole from the Spirit world. I'm here to witness this—as we all are—in this time and in this Dimension, if we so choose. God's plan is bigger than your plan or mine. The energy of love is bigger and stronger than any dark energy. All of us can choose to heal, to live in love, and witness this in the here and now.

As I trance-channel these words in the 5th Dimension, I now realize that forgiveness is the only way to salvation, especially to move forward and clear yourself and understand the healing is amazing and easy in the higher frequency of the 5th Dimension. In receiving the pain, we also receive the gifts of the Divine. If we can move the world forward in forgiveness, the negative has no power over us once we are gathered in the presence of God's light.

As you read through this book, my hope is that you are inspired to explore your own journey into the 5th Dimension. Use the stories, exercises, prayers, affirmations, and other information to lift you up and elevate your mind, body, and soul. I've arranged the book to be as user-friendly as possible, and every section was written with your upliftment in mind.

May these pages help to heal you and heal the world.

AWAKEN TO THE 5TH DIMENSION

The 5th Dimension Is . . .
Pure Love
Pure Light
Unconditional Forgiveness
Unconditional Acceptance
Instant Manifestation
Unlimited Possibilities
Beyond Time and Space
The God Vibration
Expansion
Healing
Ascension
Oneness
Interconnectedness
and so much more . . .

1

THE 5TH DIMENSION . . . AWAKENING TO YOUR OWN HIGHER CONSCIOUSNESS

Life is like riding a bicycle. To keep your balance, you must keep moving.

—ALBERT EINSTEIN

never imagined that I would one day be able to actually see through people's bodies and heal them. I am often referred to as a phenomenon because I blink in codes and receive messages from God in the 5th Dimension, where Miracles occur every day, and where the Holy Spirit is here to help us.

After my NDEs, my gifts fully awakened, but *my Spirit Guides want you to understand that you don't have to go through an NDE, or experience trauma, to find God.*

As you will realize, we not only live in a multidimensional world, we don't die. We transcend and keep raising our consciousness, if we choose to. We are all multidimensional beings with the potential to access higher Dimensions—higher states of consciousness—and because of this, we can heal ourselves faster now than ever before. Our consciousness determines what Dimension we are in at any given time and what we choose to create in our state of mind. We are nearing the Ascension and taking a clear sense of responsibility for our consciousness is absolutely necessary. Right now, I live mainly in the 5th Dimension.

Many people are experiencing the emergence of their Divine gifts as they deepen their faith and begin to live more fully in 5th Dimensional awareness and consciousness. We're witnessing people being healed quickly and more frequently. Energies are shifting. Many people thought 2012 was the end of the world; actually, it was the beginning of the Awakening. I had my NDE at the end of 2012, and at that time I knew nothing about the Mayan calendar. In that time, the supernatural of my Awakening was truly part of a vast conscious light moving into a 5th Dimensional matrix. Being a channel for Mother Mary can only come from firsthand experience. We all have abilities to tap into our own superpowers far off into a matrix of space. At this time, many Guides are here for us, to serve you and move you into the 5th Dimension, mapping the global grid.

I feel more people than ever before are ready for their own Ascension. Some feel they have had an Awakening when being healed from a severe illness or after experiencing an intimate Miracle or a Spiritual encounter. Some people have already ascended, in which they will reveal and demonstrate supernatural powers in positive ways, because we are shifting into a new energetic alignment, a 5th Dimensional level of consciousness of love and joy.

The Ascension involves calling people out on abuse, identifying abuse, correcting abuse, and letting go of abuse. If you are doing misdeeds, you're going to get caught. If you're doing good deeds, you will become known. If you have a gift, it will

become known. This is all a part of the Ascension process. The truth will be exposed, and it will be beautiful and magical.

You may wonder what exactly the 5th Dimension is and what separates it from our 3rd Dimensional material reality.

In materialist terms, scientists might describe the 3rd Dimension as where solid objects differ from two-dimensional drawings of them; whereas the 4th Dimension is space and time (time is also a Dimension that moves us forward into the 5th Dimension), and the 5th is a Dimension normally unseen by humans, which physicists believe is where gravity and electromagnetism unify.

But in spiritual terms, the 3rd Dimensional reality is artificial intelligence, electricity, technology, the glare of LED lights, suffering and pain and disease and greed and anger, and also very *me, me, me* oriented, very self-absorbed and mind-controlled. The 3rd Dimension is nonspiritual. The Guides don't like what we humans have created in the 3rd Dimensional world. They say the 3rd Dimensional world wasn't designed to exist for long because it embodies fear, egotist behaviors, and greed.

The 4th Dimension is Spirituality and love and compassion, along with the higher connections to Angels, your Guides, and the animal kingdom; while the 5th Dimension is the paranormal realm where miraculous healings come from. Many people have paranormal abilities and healing abilities in this world, but most aren't able to tune to those gifts with regularity. People can be awakened into the 5th Dimension when they begin witnessing multiple Miracles.

Let's examine these Dimensions more closely.

INTO THE REALM OF MIRACLES

Dimensions are a means of organizing different planes of existence according to their vibratory rate. Each Dimension has certain sets of laws and principles that are specific to the frequency of that Dimension. Each Dimension vibrates at a higher rate than the one below. In each higher Dimension, there exists a clearer, wider perspective of reality, a greater level of knowing. We experience more freedom, greater power, and more opportunity to create reality.

You might think that the 3rd Dimension refers to the things you see, such as the house, the tree, the animal. In this dimensional context, these things are seen as part of form, that which has shape, mass, texture, and weight. Form is also present in the 4th Dimension and to some degree in the 5th. But in these higher dimensions, things are more light-filled, not as dense as they are in the 3rd.

The 3rd Dimension is locked in time/space. This Dimension is a schoolroom that Souls attend by inhabiting humanoid physical bodies to learn more about Creation. In the 3rd Dimension, life mirrors all that we are seeking to understand. Therefore, the process of creating via our thoughts and feelings is slowed down so that we can track the circumstances of what we hold in our consciousness.

The 3rd Dimension is a state of consciousness that is very limited and restricted and dense; 3rd Dimensional society and science seek to prove that the only reality that exists is the one we perceive with our five physical senses and urges us to believe that our 3rd Dimensional perceptions of reality are the only reality. Because we've been living in this 3rd

Dimensional reality for so many lifetimes, we tend to assume that this is the only reality available to live in.

A 3rd Dimensional "operating system" runs on rigid beliefs and a fairly inflexible set of rules and limitations. For example, in the 3rd Dimension, we learn to believe that bodies are solid; they can't merge with each other or walk through walls. Everything is subject to gravity, physical objects cannot disappear, and we cannot read another person's mind. There's a solid belief that we have to work hard to accomplish our goals. Fear, judgment, and separation from the whole are pervasive.

The 4th Dimension is the bridge we're on now and will be for a relatively short period of time. In traveling through the 4th Dimension, we are preparing ourselves for the 5th. Many of us have had experiences of the 4th Dimension for a number of years now, without realizing it as we connect more to our Angelic Realm and spiritual nature. We're experiencing this Dimension when we have moments of insight and Awakening. Other times, it can happen when we're simply feeling clear and quiet inside. Everything within and around us feels lighter and less rigid.

Time is no longer linear in the 4th Dimension; 4th Dimensional perception of past, present, and future is more fluid, as the laws of time and space change. We discover that time is malleable; they can actually stretch and condense, much to our 3rd Dimensional surprise. Because of the fluid nature of time and space in the 4th Dimension, our astral forms naturally morph. Hence, there is a huge mobility of form. A shaman or holy person who can shape-shift has learned to ground their astral form upon the 4th Dimension so completely that they can temporarily change their 3rd Dimensional form.

Manifestation is much faster in the 4th Dimension. Thoughts and feelings create reality much more quickly than in the 3rd Dimension. In general, when we're experiencing love, joy, and gratitude, we're experiencing 4th Dimensional consciousness. When you have clear moments of clarity, you're in the 4th Dimension, a constant confirmation of amazing synchronicities of precious guided messages. Gratitude is the best way to live and move into the next Dimension.

The 5th Dimension is a life of Spirit, but there is still an experience of *I* as an individual member of the group. Linear time and space do not fear, and there is *no* illusion of separation or limitation. Instead, there is a constant experience of the *all*.

To enter into the 5th Dimension and stay there, all mental and emotional baggage must be left at the door. No fear, suffering, anger, hostility, guilt, or sense of separation exists there. Mastery over thought is a prerequisite.

All actions on this plane are based upon love because fear cannot survive the higher vibration of the 5th Dimension. If we were to experience fear while in the 5th Dimension, this would instantly lower us to the sub-planes of the 4th Dimension. The 5D-conscious mind has only one thing to experience, and that is love and light vibration.

5TH DIMENSION LIVING

In the 5th Dimension, we live in unconditional love, unconditional forgiveness, and unconditional acceptance. We have no fear, no hate, or judgment of any kind, or self-competition. This Dimension is where the world could and will have complete healing. In the 5th Dimension, you think about something, and it becomes present. People generally communicate through telepathy and have the ability to read each other's thoughts and feelings with ease. The experience of time is radically different; some describe it as "everything happening at once." There is no distinction between past, present, and future.

This Dimension is magical and even so crystalline, you can have superpowers. I have touched into all my clairvoyant abilities in this Dimension, and I predict many of you will be able to do the same in the near future. **This is the Dimension where healing can take place fast and easy.** It is also where many Ascended Masters are reborn into this Dimension and come back to teach here and help others, or lead people to the Awakening, which has been happening since the beginning of history.

Many of us are having experiences or dreams that feel like visits to the 5th Dimension. These are very exciting and hopeful. They keep us moving on through the difficulties that sometimes arise as we travel through the 4th Dimension and into the 5th.

Not everyone on the planet at this time is making the choice consciously, or even unconsciously, to make the shift into the 5th Dimension. All souls have the choice to enter the 5th Dimension, given they have assimilated sufficient light to hold the energy levels that exist in that higher vibration. But many will be choosing to leave the earth within several decades to move on to other 3rd Dimensional experiences in other parts of the Universe. They will not have finished with what 3rd Dimensional reality still has to teach them.

THE 5D SUPERPOWERS

Once inside the 5th Dimension, it feels like you have superpowers. Just as Superman and Superwoman gain their superpowers from Earth's yellow sun, the 5th Dimension grants us powers beyond those of normal humans. Conversely, just like kryptonite, which harms and weakens Superman and Superwoman, the 3rd Dimension drains our strength and reduces our health.

Those who are on the path of Ascension may eventually possess clairvoyance, the ability to see beyond that which is perceived with physical eyes. Clairvoyance includes seeing with the third eye, also known as the inner eye or the mind's eye. For example, words, symbols, or other information may appear in the mind's eye of a person who possesses clairvoyance. This may happen unexpectedly as a form of guidance as the person goes about their daily routine, or it may happen as a result of their own intention of going within to search for answers. Information may come regarding the person who actually possesses the ability of clairvoyance, or information that pertains to others may come through.

Those who experience clairvoyance may also see the actual unfolding of scenes in their mind's eye. The scenes play out like the scenes of a movie. They may even see objects and people moving about in the scenes, or they may see still shots of scenes. The scenes often contain pertinent information that they, themselves, may need or information that others may need.

One who possesses clairvoyance may also experience seeing the Spirits of those who have passed away. These Spirits may be higher-dimensional beings, such as Spirit Guides, or other Divine Beings, Spirits that are stuck between the 3rd Dimensional Earth and Heaven, family members who have recently departed, or other beings that are not incarnated on the 3rd Dimensional plane.

Those who experience clairvoyance may also possess the ability to see beyond the 3rd Dimensional plane. They may be able to see into the higher dimensions and into alternate realities (parallel Universes). Many parallel Universes exist in the same exact physical space that our 3rd Dimension occupies. They simply exist at an energy vibration that is different from our planetary energy vibration. Some parallel Universes exist at a higher-energy vibration than our own, and some exist at a lower-energy vibration than our planetary consciousness. Therefore, because our energy vibration does not match other energies, we normally do not perceive them.

A person who possesses the ability of clairvoyance and the other "clairs" (see below) may sometimes see into the other Universes. They may see physical objects, buildings, animals, and even other sentient beings in the other Universes. This is the opening of the third eye, the full kundalini Awakening, which happens in the 5th Dimension. After my NDE, I had all the "clairs" open up for me, including my trance channeling abilities, in the 5th Dimension.

People who possess the ability of clairvoyance may also be able to see the energy field that exists around all living things. They may see a gray energy field surrounding living things, or a gray energy field emanating from living things. They may also see an energetic duplicate of objects. Some who possess the ability of clairvoyance may even see, in great detail, the colors of the auras of others.

Once we are on the path of Ascension, the veil begins to lift, and we begin to experience our true, natural, multidimensional nature. We transition beyond the 3rd Dimension to a higher state of being. We are no longer limited to the five physical senses of the 3rd Dimension Earth plane.

In 5D terms, we each have points in our natal astrological charts that show where we can link up to 5D abilities. Our charts also show where some might be better at *using* their superhero powers than others are. What I have found to be some of the determining factors are:

1. WHICH LIFETIME YOU ARE ON OUT OF NINE IN THIS SEQUENCE OF LIFETIME STAGES OF GROWTH WITH THESE SUPERHERO POWERS.

2. IF YOU ARE UNDEVELOPED AND UNAWARE OF THEM.

3. DEVELOPED BUT UNAWARE IT IS A GIFT AND IT CREATES REACTIONS FROM OTHERS THAT MAKE IT A PERSON'S KRYPTONITE, POWERFUL WHEN IT IS USED IN POSITIVE WAYS.

4. DEVELOPING BUT UNAWARE THAT NOT EVERYONE ELSE HAS THIS POWER SO WE CAN'T UNDERSTAND *WHY* THEY DON'T GET THIS ABILITY OF OURS.

5. FULL AWARENESS OF THE POWER AND JUDICIOUS USE OF IT; GETTING IN TOUCH WITH IT AND HOW TO USE IT.

We do have these 5D abilities at our disposal. The progression of the planets has brought us to a place where we can begin to manifest them in true superhero fashion. Over the next two years, I believe we will begin to experience more awareness on a global scale with help from the higher civilizations (extraterrestrial) and Christ Consciousness.

We are now ascending in consciousness at a rapid rate into more and more 5D awareness, which will align with the Age of Aquarius. We will simply move from one Dimension to another as our own vibrational consciousness ascends higher, proving that we are multidimensional beings.

Imagine what each of these superhero powers will be like when we are *truly* like Harry Potter, living in the magic of the 5D world of love.

In a 3D time-space reality, there is a past, present, and future. All things and people are separate. This 3D reality assures that the past is always influencing the present and future. This mindset constructs, perceives, thinks, and acts according to preexisting events. This is the mind that functions according to fate. The 3D human is pushed forward in time. It evolves according to physical law and believes it is solely a body that eventually transcends.

5D humans are infinite in that they live according to universal and spiritual laws. There is no time or space. They are interconnected in the Oneness of the Universe; 5D humans understand the nature of a 3D reality yet know how to shape time and space to co-create the future. In other words, they are always, like the ancient mystics and avatars of old, dreaming their world into being. Everything, in every moment, is radically new. They have tapped the secrets of the Universe to become the creator of their destiny; 5D humans know they are Spirit as much as they exist in a body. They know they are immortal and eternal. This mindset of genius gives the 5D human a freedom from a limited life experience. They live in a 3D world, yet know how to entangle themselves in the quantum field of infinite potential of the 5th Dimension.

All dimensions and all realities exist in this moment. We create our own right to choose our own choice to live in the fastest, greatest God Frequency, the 5th Dimension. Once you learn how easy it is to get into it, you won't want to be out of it, and when you shift into the 3rd and bounce back from it and see how quickly you gain your abilities to stay in the 5th, it will become apparent you have ascended into the 5th. Depression and the negative pull of 3D no longer have to be in your existence.

The 5th Dimension is the magical Dimension within which spontaneous disappearances of cancer tumors and diseases, or genetic mutations of tissues, occur with regularity. To tap into your 5D nature, you must unlearn and un-develop the 3D mindset of the ego that separates every word, every thought, every perception in every moment.

5D humans know they are Spirit as much as they exist in a body. They know they are immortal and eternal. This mindset of genius gives 5D humans freedom from limited life experiences. They live in a 3D world, yet know how to entangle themselves in the quantum field of infinite potential of the 5th Dimension, to create a super conscious and beautifully magical life experience based exclusively on the Law of One.

THE 5TH DIMENSION'S SIX "CLAIRS"

Clairvoyance means "clear seeing."

This is when visions—past, present, and future—flash through our mind's eye, or third eye, much like a daydream. Many of us are highly visual and able to understand an idea best when we see it written or sketched out as an image on a computer screen or on a canvas. Visual people often choose to be artists, builders, photographers, decorators, designers, and so forth. If this sounds familiar, your clairvoyance is most likely a dominant sense. This helps bring out your intuition and open up your kundalini Awakening. I look at a person and can see their complete aura in a few minutes; you can also do this with practice of meditation.

Clairaudience means "clear hearing."

This is when we hear words, sounds, or music in our own mind's voice. On rare occasions, Spirit may be able to create audible sound, though this takes a tremendous amount of focused energy. Some of us retain and comprehend information best when we hear it spoken aloud. Our natural talents tend to lie in our auditory faculties, often making us gifted musicians, singers, writers, and public speakers. If this feels right to you, clairaudience may be a leading sense for you. I hear people when they cough and speak out from their throat chakra if they have certain illnesses, blocked emotional trauma, leading me into people's bodies. The breath and sound of the lungs through Spirit will give me an accurate feeling of their condition.

Clairsentience means "clear feeling."

This entails feeling a person's or Spirit's emotions or feeling another's physical pain. Many of us are clairsentient without consciously being aware of it. When we get a strong gut feeling, positive or negative, about someone we just met or when we get the chills for no apparent reason, we may be tuning in to the emotional energy of a person or a Spirit around us. When we are highly sensitive and are in tune with not only our own feelings but also the feelings of others, this makes us natural healers and caregivers. We often feel inspired to pursue careers as doctors, therapists, counselors, nannies, and teachers. If this is you, clairsentience is at the top of your senses list. This is profound. When I receive messages from the Holy Divine, I get chills, and when I find cancer or other kinds of illness, I will get hot flashes.

Clairalience means "clear smelling."

This is being able to smell odors that don't have any kind of physical source. Instances of this could include smelling the perfume or the cigarette smoke of a deceased relative, used as a sign of their presence around us. When our sense of smell is strong and distinct, we may find that certain smells connect us to past memories, or we may be drawn to working as a florist, a wine taster, or a fragrance creator. When I have a sense of different smells around, it will mean Angelic or movement of Dimensional shifts are happening.

Clairgustance means "clear tasting."

This is the ability to taste something that isn't actually there. This experience oftentimes comes from out of the blue when a deceased loved one is attempting to communicate a memory or association we have with a particular food or beverage that reminds us of them. If we have a heightened sense of taste, this would make us natural chefs, bakers, or food critics. You might have an aroma memory of your grandma making your favorite foods. Smelling the person and the food calms you as well as your loved ones from the other side.

Claircognizance means "clear knowing."

This is when we have knowledge of people or events that we would not normally have knowledge about. Spirit impresses us with truths that simply pop into our minds from out of nowhere. An example of this would be a premonition: a complete ongoing nagging warning not to do something, a forewarning of something that will happen in the future. Claircognizance requires tremendous faith because there's often no practical explanation for why we suddenly know something. Many philosophers, professors, doctors, scientists, religious and spiritual leaders, and powerful sales and business leaders tend to be highly intuitive and seem to just know the facts with a sense of certainty.

HOW TO AWAKEN YOUR HIGHER CONSCIOUSNESS

I choose to channel energies from the masters, who are here to show people how to heal themselves, how to dissolve tumors, and how to regenerate their bodies faster and permanently heal themselves when you go into a state of God Consciousness—the 5th Dimension. In the 5th Dimension, you can access Miracles and be healed instantly. We are not God but a reflection of the loving Divine feminine and masculine energy of God source Frequency. I am an energy of God, a spiritual vessel and Guide to help you transition into a higher state of consciousness. And as a trance channel, to help open your gifts.

I have been where some of you have been and where some of you are now. I, too, have experienced loss, emotional uncertainty, physical pain, illness, and heartbreak. I have experienced betrayal from family members who were supposed to be my protectors, my advocates, and my primary examples of how to give and receive love. I was in an automobile accident and suffered life-threatening injuries. I've had struggles, multiple near-death experiences, and sadness at times, but I have been healed. I could be gone right now, but I am here. We are all given challenges in this lifetime. It is important to understand that we all have lessons to learn. I am humble to know that God healed me in the 5th Dimension. I am truly grateful for this Miracle.

Prior to becoming the person I am now, I knew there were days when I did not think I would be able to make it, but I did. It is from these experiences that I now live as a light being embodiment of love, transformation, and renewal. I am deeply grateful to say I now live as spiritually strengthened living proof that even the most difficult challenges are surmountable. I share this with you so you will know no matter what you have dealt with, or are currently dealing with, you are not alone and there is hope. I am a living and breathing example of vast possibilities available to each and every one of you when you have complete faith in God and in this 5th Dimensional God Frequency. With each step you take toward personal healing, raising the vibration of your consciousness and leading by example, you create the possibility of hope.

Through my Guides, I help people awaken to their higher consciousness and activate their DNA. I am an open vessel directed to heal through my hands and scan through my eyes as I blink in multidimensional code frequencies. As I communicate through sign language and speak in 5th Dimensional Etheric Angelic Light Language, my gifts heal and awaken many people in order to help move humanity forward.

Every day, I witness miraculous healings in my office and at events I am featured. This is in a 5th Dimensional state of being. During healing events, I am divinely guided by the Holy Spirit into the audience to select several individuals to receive medical intuitive scans, revealing many diseases, emotional traumas, and unusual conditions, past and present. When the Holy Spirit Guides me to those in the group who need healing, I am told through the grace of God, through my eyes and hands, to cross their arms over their chest, then to lay on hands and heal them through Christ Light. This is the sign that the energy of the Angels and master Guides through the 5th Dimension is truly working and God has made the statement of true healing. The Guides love to invite many individuals to join me onstage to assist in the laying on of hands. This is Divine intervention and the love of the Christ Consciousness, the true Awakening of the healing of our inner life force in this magical Dimension.

When I am guided during a healing, I begin by applying holy water and anointing oil to the person's forehead and the palms of their hands. When I start to pray on the person, I often hear in my ear a gentle whisper directing me to say to them, "Do you accept the Holy Spirit?" Then the person says, "I accept the Holy Spirit." After they've had a blessing, they confirm it by saying, "I am healed."

While this is happening, the most unbelievable thing is also happening to me, which I have a hard time explaining. My body goes through a time tunnel. I feel chills, my hands are numb, and I see a lake, mountains all around, and beautiful flowers. It is so wonderful and easy. I also feel so much negative energy leaving the person's body and the person is looking up at me happy or crying with joy. Often, we say, *I am love and I am light and I am in the 5th Dimension. I am healed. I am a child of God.* The person who is on the table has been healed, set free, and looks much different. This is amazing and feels so incredible. This is when both of my eyes are blinking to signify GOD. "Hail Mary! By the power of the Divine Spirit, the person will be healed." Everything is truly being guided organically by Spirit. God wants the person to be in the 5th Dimension and to be healed, and therefore they are healed.

To help magnify the healing power in the room, the more that people witness these Miracle healings, the more we are awakened into the higher 5th Dimensional magic, like a Harry Potter movie. That is why the Holy Spirit is here more than ever in the world. Religion is not about whose God is better. When I do healings and proclaim the Holy Spirit is going through my body, this reflects the energy of God. When you tap into the energy of the Holy Spirit, you access a loving, healing vibration. The Holy Spirit is not a religion. It cannot be associated with any religion because it has nothing to do with religion. The Holy Spirit is pure love and as pure love, it is one with the energy of God. I have known this since I was a child, especially during difficult times when I felt the presence surrounding me. The meaning of God is truly love and to be healed in the world where so much suffering is happening, and yet so many Miracles at the same time makes one perhaps wonder about free will. When we take responsibility for our own actions and consciousness, we win, and that's when we move forward. We rise up and raise each other up. Our struggles are our strengths. Forgiveness is painful but possible and necessary to not accumulate unwanted energy of the 3rd Dimension.

Healing is one of the most important things you can learn and experience in life. It teaches you how to become involved in your own personal outcome and the outcome of others. It extends to the personal actions and choices you make for your free will and your well-being and the well-being of others. Considering that we are living in 3rd Dimensional unprecedented times, we need unprecedented healing tools—supplemental and 5th Dimensional spiritual tools that teach us how to strengthen our bodies, minds, and Spirits. Healing is multifaceted. It encompasses the spiritual, mental, and emotional body as well as the physical. When we have the right tools, the highest tools, to actively participate in our own healing, we can move forward to heal ourselves.

During private sessions, I relay supplemental informational tools to further support all aspects of healing by addressing topics that include self-protection tools, Awakening your God Consciousness, organic holistic living and nutrition, boosting your immune system, avoiding toxic exposure to mercury and plastics, exclusive information about water, dechlorinating shower filters, meditation, and daily prayer.

In addition to supplemental tools and learning how to survive in a 3rd Dimensional world while building an intimate relationship with the 5th Dimensional frequency of God Consciousness, spiritual tools also include Awakening your highest gifts through DNA activation and telomeres, the protective caps on DNA strands that shorten with age and bad dietary habits. By lengthening your telomeres with a healthy diet and meditation, you can enhance your health and lifestyle.

When my Guides use me to do DNA activation through your eyes, it allows for a transmission and an easier progression into 5th Dimensional consciousness. At the time you experience a change in your DNA, it begins to awaken the body as the result of growth that is now underway. One of the ways to activate the body is through the eyes, and we can experience a Christ Consciousness Awakening through our DNA being activated. Through the transmission of eye contact, I channel activations, and you may have an enlightenment through your eyes. DNA activation is a wonderful healing tool that can be used to remove sabotaging beliefs and experiences that can become lifelong impediments. When the Guides do the DNA eye activations, you can leave the 3rd Dimension and you start to awaken to your full potential—your gifts from birth. The trauma leaves your DNA, and you can have a rebirth. (This exercise is explained in the DNA activation chapter.) The full enlightenment of the trauma pattern woven into your brain, and kept locked into the "computer," can be released and you can move into a higher GOD Consciousness. The world is much easier and lighter. The frequency moves with you. The 3rd Dimension is now harder for you, and you are drawn into a state of a faster pull of rhythm and telomeres, which is good for longevity of life span.

CONSCIOUSNESS IN THE 5TH DIMENSION

By understanding we can embrace the 5th Dimension consciousness, we can fill our body with trust, love, and the light. It is through the grace of God's loving energy that our DNA can be healed and pain can be turned into light. God is energy. We all have the ability to tap into this energy, manifest it, and receive it into our bodies. It's quite simple when you learn how to release 3rd Dimensional energy, because healing can't happen in the 3rd Dimension. The 3rd Dimension is where disease, pain, and suffering reside.

The 5th Dimension is magical. It is where we come from. The energy of the 5th Dimension is a perfectly balanced duality of feminine and masculine energy. And when you start to go into this Dimension, the 5th Dimension—the Divine Consciousness, it's a ride! When you're on this ride, while I am laying hands on you and healing you of a particular disease, hernia, ailment, or even cancer, and your hands are held up high or in prayer on your heart chakra while you are channeling with me, feeling and truly accepting the love light energy as it dissolves out of your body, the energy is truly of a higher 5th Dimension, and it is amazing. The Energy of God is an actual energy that you feel during the healing, and this can be experienced in a webinar or huge stadium; nothing is too vast for the Holy Spirit. Scalar Energy and God can travel through all space and time.

Despite the challenges of living in the density of 3rd Dimensional energies, my Guides are saying it is time to move forward. The time for dwelling on past hurts, resentments, disappointments is past, and emotional karmas are gone when we move into a 5D state of mind. This is the time of the Ascension, the time for individual and collective physical and spiritual healing, and expansion of consciousness. The time has come to let go of the belief that to have spiritual and personal growth you have to linger in suffering. This is a false belief, and false conditioning, which have been held on to for long enough.

I believe in the next few years, more and more people will

have a full Awakening. The world is shifting more rapidly, and the good news is because of the 5th Dimensional teachings, the healings will become wiser and more knowledgeable. There will be a 5D organic living lifestyle with 5D foods and 5D spiritual relationships, which will move all of us together into this Awakening. So it is important for us to stay in this magical God Frequency as we shift together.

Everyone can bring in the highest Spirit Guides and the highest Angels. You can be a spiritual warrior and turn your scars into triumphs. You can turn emotional wounds into glorious multidimensional progress to heal yourself and the world. With high spiritual energies available to everyone, more and more people are going to massively be healed. Every day, my body holds more light and more energy from the masters. This allows me to become stronger as a trance channeler and medical intuitive. In my work and in my life, I am constantly moving forward, and I am living proof of what is possible through God.

People often ask me why I was chosen to do this work. It is the soul within me that has reincarnated to help people move into the Ascension. *When in the flow of doing my service, I feel a joyful, ecstatic exuberance.* I transform the energy of people's bodies, which is why I am called an alchemist. I do this as an agent of God. I do the work I am directed to do.

As a spiritual form, in existence and chosen many times before, this soul chose to do this work before I was born. I feel many people here have been chosen and are going to see soon they are healers and gifted in many ways to serve with Spirit. This is a joyful way to help the transition through our Awakening. If people make themselves available to let in their Guides and Angels, and not let in 3D fear, and stay in the 5th Dimension, and equally care about the inner and outer spiritual world, and learn new tools related to spiritual ways of being, we can gain peace through kindness, as Dr. Martin Luther King Jr. proclaimed, and we all can take part in healing our world.

It is my hope that you fully embrace the idea that Spirituality can be an invaluable part of your life. God can be a part of your life. Our world does not have to be loud and angry. We can be peaceful, loving, and calm.

My Guides are highly intellectual, yet deeply compassionate for you and humanity, and they are saying, "We have arrived."

Who I am, and my gifts, being a trance channel, and my Guides, come from higher civilizations. "We are messaging. We are here."

They have arrived to tell people to spread joy and excitement so that we can move into the highest state of 5th Dimensional healing.

2

FINDING HEALING IN THE 5TH DIMENSION

*S*imilar to surgical hands-on healing, with laying on hands, I am in the presence of God and am completely taken over by Spirit. It is not me who is doing the work. It is the Spirit of God working through me as a vessel in the 5th Dimension.

When I lay hands on a person's throat, I often see a lot of negative energy, but it can immediately move off the throat with the permission of the client and acceptance of the Holy Spirit. Negative energy can attach to you on any part of your body when you are upset, and it then can develop into disease. This is the energy that can formulate into a tumor, throat cancer, or perhaps issues of the thyroid.

ALIGNING YOURSELF WITH GOD

It's important to be 100 percent in alignment with God and not breathing out your anger, or the anger directed toward you from someone else. This is how negative energy can become trapped inside the body. Remember, don't take on others' negative energy, because it could be they are being attacked also. You can stay in your higher self and counter it with love and stop the negative with forgiveness and embracing God. Please know this is vital so you don't take on physical ailments.

It's important to have yourself aligned and committed to a God Consciousness frequency so when you're attacked by a negative energy from a lower frequency, you can be fully protected to release that negative energy through your breath. Because we're multidimensional beings, we have the choice and the power to live in the God Frequency.

To illustrate, let's say you work in a retail store and experience an angry customer who screams and yells at you. As a result, you feel angry and frustrated and depressed. This negative energy directed at you, now internalized as negative emotions, can then become trapped inside your body. A lot of people get sick and blame themselves for getting sick, internalizing guilt and interpreting the manifestation of disease as their fault.

There needs to be clarification that no one can be completely conscious of everything going on at all times. Since you are not 100 percent conscious of everything going on around you all the time, you are going to breathe in negative energy; therefore, it's really essential to be as close to 100 percent in faith with God's energy, the 5th Dimensional Realm where Miracles happen. Although we cannot be consciously aware of all the negative energy around us at all times, you can choose to be conscious of yourself. When you remain 100 percent in faith with the energy of God and use deep breathing out of the solar plexus to purge negative energy, and are more aware of your surroundings, you are more likely to not breathe in and hold on to negative energy. (These 5th Dimensional exercises are explained in this book.)

When we are in touch with our breath throughout the day, engaging in deep breathing, we can know that we are love and light. We can call in the Holy Spirit and breathe out negative energy while knowing that disease is an energy that can be released. Illness is an energy that enters the body, and it is an energy that can be removed from the body. If we remain within the presence of God throughout the day, healing is absolutely possible. (I explain how later in this book.)

When someone comes to me for a private healing session or attends one of my healing events, they must be open and truly want to be healed through the energy of the Holy Divine. They can still have doubts or fears about being healed, but once the healing begins, their fear disappears because they have entered into a 5th Dimensional state of consciousness, and a frequency of love. They turn their fears into love, and this helps them to accept their own higher consciousness.

When I first began to pray on my head to heal myself, there first had to be a belief that healing was possible. This cannot be emphasized enough. When a person comes for healing and has a tumor(s), but is not 100 percent in faith with God, I can feel them fighting and resisting the healing because they are not breathing in enough oxygen. God is energy and oxygen. You are made of oxygen and created by light; therefore, if you would have a scan with me, I would instruct you to keep breathing and connecting with God and light. As long as you are breathing deeply during the scan, I can more easily pick up on the energy inside you.

During the scan, when I am channeling the source of God and light to review your entire body, you are also channeling the source of God and light. Ultimately, we all are energy. As the vessel, I am an agent for God, the Christ Consciousness, and the person. During the healing, we are in the 5th Dimension. If there is an internal struggle within the person to let go and receive, I feel the struggle. I also feel when the person lying on the table has been beaten down, feels defeated, and has simply given up. A person in this state will not wholeheartedly fight the negative energy to leave their body while I pray. When I feel their struggle, I help the person by giving chants so they can feel safe with God to express their prayer. It can be any prayer. It does not have to be religious. For example, a prayer could be, "I am love, I am light," or calling in the simple chant of Om. But the person must have the will to do it.

When the negative energy begins to leave, I feel the energy depart, as well as when it is finally released. It is absolutely heaven in the highest. I see Miracles every day, and the magic is God. The client must let themselves go into the 5th Dimension and awaken to their healing and open to their gifts. At this point, many have tried everything and this was their last recourse for healing.

To watch a tumor dissolve in front of me is unexplainable, at least on the human level, yet explainable on the spiritual level because it is God. If you were to ask me why, or how this is happening, my answer is this is the energy of God and the Holy Spirit. Heaven is here. We can, in fact, heal our entire bodies and heal the entire planet, our minds are so powerful. Our own gifts are often opened through understanding that what we loved the most, when we were young and passionate about it, was Spirit telling us this was one of our gifts.

THE HOLY SPIRIT AND YOU

The Holy Spirit is our higher consciousness, an energy that we can all tap into. It is all that is good, honest, and pure. When you tap into this energy and trust it, it is so powerful that you can awaken your intuition and open to your gifts, healing any disease, surmounting any obstacle or physiological cellular disruption. It is the absolute Righteous Light.

I call in the 5th Dimension by stepping into this daily practice with my Ascension into the 5th Dimension channeled prayer, which can help many people to stay centered and awakened. (See it later in this book.) Many people are reaching this powerful energy. I speak to God through my eyes, and God has told me to call in the Holy Spirit through prayer or meditation, anchored in the heart. Meditation can also call in the Holy Spirit and the Divine. Any prayer that calls through the heart will summon the higher source of love, no matter what your faith, religion, or belief. As a powerful energy and honorable to you when you surrender over to it, it will flow through your body and completely heal you. Every minute of the day, you can call in the power of the Divine. I will be showing you ways to do this.

People ask me, "I pray a lot. Why are my needs not being met?"

With this question, I hear a lot of emphasis placed on "I want." What about "I shall not want?" I respond, "We are never to say, 'I want.'" The fact that "I want" is the basis of so many prayers indicates that somewhere, something has gone off track.

The person then usually responds with, "Well, how should I speak? How should I pray?"

The relationship with God should be one of give-and-take, which includes gratitude, love, and respect. You work *with* the energy of God. It is not about "I want." It doesn't work this way. God should always be honored and loved. God hears our prayers every moment of the day. When we are not honoring and loving God, we are listening to another energy. That is how intimate the relationship is with God. There is only one path. God is an energy that is strong with commitment and honor. When you witness as many Miracles as I have witnessed, you honor the glory of the Miracle. I've included powerful 5D prayers for you in a later chapter in this book.

When people come for a healing event or office visit, they raise both hands to say, "I accept the Holy Spirit. I'm going into the 5th Dimension," and through this acceptance of the Holy Spirit, you can be healed. My Guides want hundreds of people to proclaim this in unison. They want people to honor the energy, the Holy Spirit, and declare love for God. Sometimes, to my surprise, it sounds as if we are going back to the days of old-school faith healing, but this is needed. The Guides are directing me as they move through me since my NDEs, during this time of a fast and grand transition. When you have large groups of people gathered with pure intention to call in the Holy Spirit, shifts take place at a much faster rate.

The Holy Spirit is a heart connection that immediately brings God back into the world. The Guides want you now to be awakened through the Holy feminine Divine in the 5th Dimension to love your brothers and sisters, never to judge another, and to serve. By doing these things, you can be activated by your Guides. The more you witness the miraculous Miracles, the more we shift into this higher state of super consciousness. As our thoughts shift and transform faster and are no longer stuck in a pain-related 3D world, we will see more of our own faster spontaneous healing take place. It is the power of science and God in the 5D world. Your body, like mine, is rewired to go beyond the supernatural. My DNA activation exercises and meditations have shifted many thousands of people because they have seen Miracles through the Guides and the Holy Divine.

THE MIRACLES AND YOUR ACTIVATION

My Guides want people to be activated now to awaken their gifts. When I am at events, I invite family members or loved ones to come up onto the stage to participate in the healing of their loved one. My Guides want the energy of Divine light to pass through their hands. I once did a healing on a man who attended an event with his four small children. When he was selected by my Guides to come up for healing, as his four children stood beside him, he lay on the table and they placed their hands on him and prayed with him when I began the healing.

I can teach people how to generate the power of the Holy Divine through their bodies. They can feel the energy come through them while they lay hands on the person and we pray. You can feel the energy! You can feel it happening. You can see it! The prayer can be anything, like "I am love, I am light." More people gathered with good intentions generate more power. It is amazing when you watch the Miracles. A lot of people witnessing the healing start to cry, confirming it with emotion. My Guides like when people join together, when everyone and their souls can be gathered in unity as one. It's something that the whole room can feel. When gathered together, it's called a superpower 5th Dimensional grid.

When everyone accepts the Holy Divine, we will no longer have suffering in the world. If everyone would accept each other, the negative energy would leave our entire Universe. Imagine what would happen if the world understood that healing cancer can escape the moneymaking cancer industry because the healing energy of God is free. Everything is energy. Again, illness is an energy in the body that can leave the body.

Raising your vibration fills your body more with God. Because I healed myself through God, I believe we all can heal ourselves. We can have a love revolution with God as our healer. We can live in Christ Consciousness, a loving 5th Dimensional consciousness, right now. It is up to each and every one of us to choose the direction in which we want our lives and our world to go.

By helping others to heal and witnessing their healing, you, too, can be healed by the power of the Holy Spirit. For you to experience this realm where Miracles are made and profound healing happens, you only need to open your mind and your heart to your own endless spiritual potential.

As an open vessel, I receive healing codes from many Divine energy forms, guided by a feedback system where I blink and use my hands to perform psychic surgery so disease in the body disappears in the 5th Dimension. My Guides are my teachers.

God is energy. God is love. We all have the ability to tap into this energy, manifest it, and receive it into our bodies. It is through the energy of love and light that the body can heal. I believe that to receive the love of God's energy, you truly need the commitment of having, as the saying goes, "both feet in," meaning to have full commitment. The image of one foot in and one foot out leaves room for a person to be an open vessel for negative energy to enter the body. It is about you making a commitment to the Universe, the light, and God with both feet in.

Some of the tools to use in keeping both feet in include blessing your food and walking away from any angry situation. Chanting positive prayers, sound vibrations, loving each other, not judging, staying in a higher consciousness, and keeping two feet in God's loving energy—this is how we move mankind forward.

The prayers and practices in this book will help you to stay fully committed, with both feet in!

CHANNELING, BLINKING, AND GOD

I am constantly channeling, and some people call me the blinking-walking channeler. I go into a deeper channel, a sound tunnel where I hear ocean waves. I look off and I start blinking faster, like I am blind, and there are fast white lights flashing at me. I see and I pick up more spiritual Guides when this is happening. I ask the client to fill themselves with love and light and to keep breathing and relax. It's fascinating, like having a scientific spiritual MRI or X-ray. The more they inhale and exhale, I pick up on all the energy faster. I blink and scan my hands over them, detecting everything across their bodies. I also can be guided to blink how many years back an injury or condition happened to them.

I am guided by the Holy Spirit and given sign language with my hands tapping my body and the client's body, getting more information about their detailed body assessments. Then I feel like a puppet who's being moved by the most amazing energy in this Universe. The surgical healings I do are very intense. The Holy Spirit, Jesus, and Mother Mary come right through my hands, my hands start kneading away, feeling like they are in a pair of gloves. When they heal a person, I am taken over as a complete vessel, and I obey God.

The left eye blinking means things are completely good and healthy. The right eye blinks when things are not good. Both eyes blink together when there is a God-significant occurrence like an accident, surgery, or NDE where the Divine Energy has come in to save you. I ask some people, "Have you had an accident or had an NDE?" It usually takes them a minute or two, but it clicks, and they remember. So, at that point, they know they were, and are, saved by the Spirit.

Now that I have been upgraded by Spirit, people don't necessarily have to formulate yes or no questions. I can answer them directly from the Divine.

The whole healing is guided by my blinking while my hands are numb and scanning. The right eye starts blinking to perform the surgery and to pinpoint the issue. The left eye begins processing the Spirit into the body, meaning you are accepting the healing. Both eyes start blinking to say Spirit has healed your body.

I believe the Holy Spirit is one with God. The Oneness is pure Divine Energy, an omnipotent energy that I believe can create all, heal all, be all, and constitutes our entire Universe.

I feel that we all can tap into the higher state of consciousness. The higher thoughts and consciousness, they are God, the good, loving thoughts. It's when you can naturally open up the third eye and the crown chakra, open up to the Divine energy of God, and surrender to the higher dimensions, knowing that we can be safe in that energy and stay in that energy. We can all be peacemakers in this world and take responsibility to call in this higher Christ Consciousness.

Everybody has a different spiritual Awakening process. For some people, it happens very fast; for some, it takes a lifetime to reach Awakening. I have seen some people who have taken many classes on how to be more spiritual, and others who have never been to such a class and still have their Awakening.

Each person will have his or her own Awakening at their own speed and in their own time.

I am able to detect trapped emotions and negative energies and direct light energy into those areas, but unless the person's thought pattern is changed, those same emotions will come back and again trigger disease. Because we are made up of energy, keeping negative emotions in the body for too long can cause disease. The higher your dimensional consciousness, the harder it is for negative energy to be in your cells. Love is a healing energy and the strongest weapon we have.

When you sense negative energy inside of you, feel it, then breathe it out while saying, **"I am love, I am light."** Always call on your own Guides and ask for help. We have many Guides. It can be a lover who has passed, or an Angelic being, or one who has been with you since birth. When you need help, call on them and listen for their response. That is why they are here, to assist you.

If you wonder if Miracles happen, if tumors can dissolve, if cancer can disappear, I say, ABSOLUTELY! And you can say ABSOLUTELY!

I will show in this book ways that I've learned to awaken your gifts by using your Spirituality to heal yourself through the God Frequency.

Being a Medium, I feel this is the truth: we are NOT ALONE! We are always connected to God Consciousness, a third-eye Awakening. But we need to honor this so we can move into a super conscious reality. We all can have superpowers when tapping into this 5th Dimensional Realm. We not only can change our health with astronomical results, like healing cancer and any physical or emotional conditions, but these are miraculous Miracles we cannot take all the credit for. This is where we say, "I am a child of God," and accept the healing in the 5th Dimensional God Frequency.

If Jesus and many other Ascended masters were alive today, they would be doing their work in the 5th Dimension.

MYSTICAL EXPERIENCES HEIGHTEN 5D AWARENESS

There are four states of consciousness: **wakefulness, sleeping, dreaming, and the transcendental.** The transcendental state of consciousness is a state of awareness that is often associated with mystical experiences, and it's the mystical that allows us to experience another aspect of the self.

To say this another way, this means we have to *transcend* the known self to experience some other aspect of our *potential* unknown self. To get beyond the known self is what begins to fill in the mystery of the self, and that moment awakens us to our journey back to source. In other words, there is more to you than meets the eye.

In the case of the mystical, the experience comes not from an external world, it comes from an internal one. When you have a mystical, transcendental experience, it is as if your senses heighten to such a degree that the internal experience causes you to become more aware of the 5D experience.

Let's delve into the 5th Dimension Life a little more deeply . . .

3

THE 5TH DIMENSION PATH OF LIFE

Life's most persistent and urgent question is,
"What are you doing for others?"

—MARTIN LUTHER KING JR.

've been healed today in the 5th Dimension!" I often
hear this declaration made after many have experienced
the 5th Dimension.

The 5th Dimension is real and accessible to everyone.
In the 5th Dimension, it is possible to heal at a level that most
people and scientists would consider Miracle healings. However, they only seem to be Miracles because we have so little

understanding of the 5th Dimension and how we can access it to heal us, here in our present reality.

By witnessing Miracles, you can become more open to experiencing your own Miracle. The more you are being of service, the more you can raise your consciousness. By raising our hand in service to others, this is how we shift the planetary consciousness.

How can you recognize the presence of God Consciousness when we're in the 5th Dimension? How can you live successfully in the 3rd Dimension?

LIVING BEYOND WORRY AND FEAR

We are multidimensional beings living in a multidimensional world. Anything that feels positive, loving, and kind is rooted in the higher consciousness of God and the Holy Spirit. Anything that feels shameful, angry, worrisome, fearful, or hateful is a negative consciousness, which is not of God and the Holy Spirit.

You may also wonder how to recognize the presence of God amid worry. Worry is an aspect of the human condition that is sometimes difficult to avoid. From an energetic perspective, worry blocks almost everything, except more of that which you do not want. When you engage in excessive worry, your energy is heavy and sluggish. This low vibration of the energy makes it extremely difficult, if not impossible, for the higher energies to reach your consciousness. Even though you may want assistance with whatever it is you are dealing with, and you long for spiritual help, when you remain in deep and excessive worry, you become the biggest impediment to receiving the helping gifts from God.

In this worrisome state of lower 3rd Dimensional consciousness, which many people currently vibrate to, you cannot always recognize the presence of God because your attention and awareness are focused on the problem and not the solution. Living in this world makes it unavoidable for us to engage in some level of worry. You can, however, worry minimally and let it pass. You must not allow yourself to worry for weeks and months on end, because prolonged worry results in your energy remaining stagnant, in low vibration, preventing you from spiritual progress. You will instead attract more unwanted circumstances in alignment with the low frequency of your vibration. Simply put, like attracts like; low vibration attracts low vibrational experiences.

Alternatively, when you sincerely surrender and turn your fears and worries over to God, you allow the energy to begin to flow. You can receive what God wants for you. Let's be clear, surrender does not mean to give up. Surrender means that you act from a place of pure faith and trust that God will consciously move you toward the highest outcome. Consciousness is designed for solutions; when you raise your vibration to a higher level of consciousness, you fill your body more with the presence of God. By allowing yourself to remain open to receive *soul*-utions, you will have more of an intimate relationship with God and ultimately, with your Higher Self.

Since high vibration attracts high vibrational experiences, you have to utilize spiritual tools so you don't fall back into the darkness of the 3rd Dimension. You can't say, "I'm in with

God," and then go into a store and yell at someone, then try to rationalize your outburst by saying you were tested. The high-vibrational relationship with God and yourself is one of the most important tools to maintain a high consciousness.

THE PRESENT MOMENT AND MIRACLES

Let me further clarify why most people continue to ask, "How can I be more connected to God? How can I know that God exists? How can I have more of an intimate relationship with God?"

These types of questions tell me that most people live in an unconscious state of existence. It means **that if you are constantly looking for something other than what you have, you are not living in the present moment.** Living in the present moment allows you to see the utterly miraculous that happens around us all the time. To stay in the present moment and create an intimacy with your God Consciousness, focus mindfully on your breath. The inner freedom comes from learning how to balance thoughts and the present moment as a multidimensional being, staying un-attached to the present moment.

A Miracle is an event that is inexplicable by natural or scientific laws, because it is rooted in a higher consciousness of God and the Holy Spirit. However, the miraculous can reveal itself in many ways, such as stabilized health, renewed relationships, unexpected forgiveness, timely abundance, guidance, or answered prayers, all for which gratitude can and should be expressed. If you're looking for a specific representation of what you think God or Miracles should consist of, or resemble, you will continually miss the signs that indicate the presence of God and the Holy Spirit.

To have an intimate relationship with God Consciousness, and stay healed, comes by spreading the word of God. You can't be healed with the energy of the Holy Spirit and go back to your old ways. Period! At the close of each of my healing sessions with clients, I ask them to touch the area that has been healed. When you touch the place on your body where healing has occurred, this touch signifies your acceptance and proclamation of being healed. The physical contact of your hand with the healed area further declares and affirms the healing.

Unfortunately, many people who have been healed fail to continue proclaiming their healing. Some leave one of my Healing Trilogy events, or my office after a private session, and go on with their life as usual. These individuals forget about what they have received. They don't give testimonials to others who may need or want to hear what they have experienced, nor do they express any thoughts of how they can circulate the goodness of what they have received. Placement of your hand on your body where healing occurred is one way to declare what has been received, but it isn't the only way.

Gratitude can be extended out into the world in the form of volunteerism, compassion, or altruism. There is a bigger picture demonstrated by those who proclaim their healing and give testimonials, not solely on video at one of the healing events but in their social circles and among loved ones. Social media can be used as a positive influence, especially with so much pain and negativity in the world today; people need to see and hear about what is possible through God. When you put your trust into the Holy Divine, it expands and there is no better person to relay this message than one who has received. Declare your healing every day so that you remember it and help others.

LET GO OF FEAR

Releasing fear is one of the most important things you can do for yourself, and love is the answer. Fear is often defined as an unpleasant emotion. Whether it's real or imagined, it can hold you back.

In the traditional sense, the primary purpose of fear is to preserve life. Primordial fears and anger that were once a part of everyday life—such as fear of being eaten alive by a vicious predator—are no longer as prevalent as they once were; much of the fear we associate with simply staying alive has been pacified, but the way in which we use fear has intensified. From persuasion, to manipulation and control, we have been conditioned to listen to anything and anyone but our own inner intuitive voice. We have become a fear-based society that uses fear to drive most of the decisions, policies, and agendas that are kept in place.

Fear of someone, or something, maintains such an apparent grip on the collective psyche that it no longer seems out of place. Fear signifies and perpetuates a belief that you are not safe and that you cannot let down your guard; that you must protect yourself at all times because self-preservation is of the most importance. This way of being can only be experienced within the 3rd Dimensional energy, in which every single person has learned how to live and function within the energy of fear.

Fortunately, the time of living and co-creating from a place of fear is no longer being energetically supported. With the miraculous healings and Awakenings that are taking place, we are beginning to see what is possible when we access higher consciousness. You cannot uphold the healing energy of the Holy Spirit if your energy remains attached to the fear associated with the 3rd Dimension. The fear, whether it's personal or collective, has to be released.

When you let go of fear (see the New 5th Dimension Way of Healing exercise to release fear), you will not be triggered by outside circumstances and global scare tactics, nor will you let other people trigger you. You will know that there is no need to overanalyze a situation in anticipation of the worst possible outcome. You will understand that you do not need to try to control and manipulate outcomes to feel safe. You are eternally tethered to God. As your consciousness rises, you will come to truly understand and know there is nothing to fear. With God as your anchor, you will come to find the spiritual freedom that can only be found in fearlessness.

BE IN YOUR BODY

When you're grounded in your body, this is the most powerful way to connect with the energy of the 5th Dimension. When you are in your body, you're quiet. We reside mostly in our thinking mind so it is easy to dissociate from the body. When you are grounded in your body, you can hear inner guidance and you are less judgmental of yourself and others, and you move into your heart more. Breathing through the emotional pain of your human experience makes more room for your soul to inhabit your body. That helps you to ground.

In this state of being connected to your body, you're less vulnerable to the external chaos of 3rd Dimensional energies. When you aren't grounded, your energy feels unstable, like a leaf blown about in the wind. Being grounded and settled within yourself allows your consciousness to be connected with the earth and the presence of God. Like a tree firmly rooted amid a storm, some leaves and branches may be affected, but the core of the tree stands firmly in place.

Being in your body lifts your awareness out of compulsive, fear-based thinking. When you're caught up in your mind, your attention and energy are scattered like leaves blown off the tree. When you're in the present moment with your breath, your energy is tethered within and you're more aware.

The more effective way to connect with the reality of the present moment is when you're connected to your breath, because the stream of thoughts grows more quiet. With fewer thoughts passing through your awareness, you become more receptive to what is trying to reach you and more available to meet the 5th Dimensional energies. (Note: Many of the exercises in the upcoming chapters will help ground you in your body.)

LOVE FREELY

The only way for us to love freely is to let the love that already exists in our hearts flow effortlessly. You can do this by practicing good communication, expressing your feelings honestly, and giving unconditional love, which requires not placing any conditions on how you accept another person. It requires the strength to set personal boundaries, but the ability to still fully accept everyone with an open heart. This is a pure example of God's love. Our natural state is to be in a state of unconditional love, but we have moved away from our true nature. We spend too much time and energy protecting our hearts. Despite the illusions of suffering that we have attached to our experience of love, we need to relinquish the negative perceptions we have about giving and receiving it.

By putting protection around your heart, you prevent love from flowing freely. Love is always ready and wants to flow effortlessly between people, but we have to choose to let go of the fear so this energy can flow in and out of our hearts. We are meant to embody love. When we do not give and receive unconditional love, we can feel that something important to our survival is missing. We operate defensively, all the while longing for love.

When we step into the place of being willing to love unconditionally, the love flows freely and we embody unity. When we allow energy to flow in and out of our hearts, we realize it is not love that hurts. Unconditional love for ourselves and others is our natural state when we vibrate higher throughout our bodies and our souls, and we can project other loving situations to us. We can project love onto all aspects of the world, and in this state, the entire world can be raised as we picture the planet Earth in complete peace and harmony. To maintain high consciousness and remain connected to the healing energy of the Holy Spirit, letting down barriers to love is essential.

DISCOVERING SELF-ACCEPTANCE

If you're on a serious mission for spiritual and personal growth, there is no self-judgment to be made. To be awakened in this human form, you cannot judge yourself or others, because we are all at the right space and time. We are not here to make enemies and pass judgments, and there are no mistakes. Because we are human, we are here to learn about ourselves.

We all have gifts that are specific to our earthly life experience. It's self-judgment that prevents us from moving into our gifts, purpose, and commitment to the Holy Spirit. You are here to awaken through your human form. One part of the Awakening is the acceptance of who you are in this human form because there is something you came here to do. A good example of this is my life and the difficulty I had in letting go of the life I wanted to live to accept the life I was meant to live.

As a healer, I have not always wanted to accept who I am. Some time ago, I spoke with a close friend who said to me, "I don't know who you are anymore. You talk, walk, and look differently than you used to. You're doing things you never used to do. You cry sometimes because you don't like all the ways your life has changed. I wonder, who are you? And even though I don't fully know who you are, I do know that you have to accept who and what you are. You should be used to all of this change by now."

Once I got to the point in my life when I could look in the mirror and truthfully say, "I accept you. I accept you. I accept who I am now," I would blink to confirm. From that point on, every time I thought of myself and the newness of my healing gifts and life as I had come to know it, and said, "I accept you," I began to feel better and more gifts began to open up for me. In addition to self-acceptance, I also had to undergo a period of balancing the feminine and masculine energies within me that had worked against each other.

The left side of your body relates to the feminine aspect of your consciousness; the right side of your body relates to the masculine aspect. We need the feminine energy to be present and strong in ourselves and across the planet right now. For so long, the dominance of male energy and consciousness has remained in the forefront of our personal lives, and this imbalance of the feminine and masculine energy has caused internal and external conflict on many levels, affecting each and every one of us, including me.

For years, a part of me did accept who I am now and what I'm doing, but it wasn't full acceptance. These parts of ourselves must be in balance because they represent both aspects of the Holy Spirit, which is one and all, encompassing both energies. As I said "I accept you," I felt as if I was being healed through balancing the feminine and masculine aspects of my consciousness. Self-acceptance is a vital tool that continues to help me fully tap into higher consciousness. When we accept both the feminine and the masculine, this begins to calm the overbearing aspect of the masculine energy and creates an opening for balance to be felt, accepted, and integrated on a personal and internal level, so it can then manifest on the external, global level.

Women have been encouraged to act more male oriented and to develop the masculine aspect of themselves to survive in this culture. Women have used this energy to get the right to vote, to fight back after being beaten down mentally or physically, to find productive and meaningful work, to raise strong children, and ultimately, to survive. However, we don't have to continue using forceful energy in the same way that we did in the past to be strong in this world, even if this has previously been the way of the world.

We are no longer of the time when the male perspective has to determine what feminism, womanhood, personal strength, leadership, and power will encompass. We can be strong, loving, and empowered peacemakers. We don't have to be strong with dominance and force.

My life is proof that you can indeed be a powerful, strong, and effective leader who stands in love of the Divine feminine and makes decisions from a place of love. Despite the challenges many of us face, including my own, we can still go and do the work of God as our calling from a strong and powerful place within ourselves. Regardless of whether you are a man or a woman, there is a place for both masculine and feminine energy to work together in Christ Consciousness. The voice of the peacemaker who walks this new energy into existence to heal our planet, our bodies, and our souls can do this in a loving way and still be heard.

THE POWER OF FORGIVENESS

Forgiveness is the key and the energy of loving deeply through our wounded hearts. After my near-death experience, I felt a complete release for the people who had harmed me through my early years. Forgiveness is a muscle; the more you use it, the stronger it gets. Try to forgive as many people as you can, because when they harmed you, it was in their 3rd Dimensional consciousness, a lower state of consciousness. If they'd had a higher God Frequency, they would have never abused you.

Letting this energy go brings you such great freedom and raises your frequency. Holding grudges lowers your vibration and keeps you trapped in the 3rd Dimension, causing sickness to your emotional and physical body. The pain release is so important so we don't carry anxiety, yet to think of forgiving perpetrators can be hard when we have been so deeply wounded. The more we practice compassion in forgiving others, the more we dig deep in our souls and the lighter the world starts to feel around us, and we see a higher vibrational love.

When letting go, remember to release the past, let go of the what-ifs in life, stop beating yourself up, and most importantly, forgive.

If you have a relative, friend, coworker, or love relationship who is abusive toward you, this can be extremely challenging.

Just remember it is not your fault because they are in a 3rd Dimensional energy and they have their own percentage of consciousness, and the abuser could have had other circumstances that led them into a darker energy. I can understand your tears and how hard it is to move through it. You can set yourself free; you are not them, your karma is not their karma. You did not inherit their genes, and you are you. You are special.

I know the Miracles are in the 5th Dimension, but you can forgive them in the 3rd Dimension and break the cord. In forgiving it sets you free, and even if the cellular memory might still be there, the DNA energy is gone. I forgave them so you can forgive them.

See Part Two for a powerful 5th Dimension forgiveness exercise.

3RD AND 5TH DIMENSIONAL RELATIONSHIPS

Our 3rd Dimensional relationships were built to break. Our job as 3rd Dimensional human beings was to experience separation, loss, and fear. Humanity agreed to participate in this Divine experiment of amnesia, requiring our civilization to find its way back to the source of its own free will. We learned to destroy connection rather than honor it, to the point that we were in danger of destroying our civilization and the world in which we lived.

5th Dimensional relationships are built to sustain themselves. They eternally exist within the context of Creation, and their experience on the Earth plane is one of reconnection with our Divine nature, the essence of our being. Your 5th Dimensional soul family supported your journey on Earth through an ignorant human mind, by providing you with a group of beings who incarnated with you over and over again. Known as your soul group, these individuals played different familial and community roles over your multiple incarnations, always supporting your growing evolutionary awareness that there is more to life than fear and pain. Because your human mind could not conceive the soul connections continually supporting it, you felt abandoned, alone, and often emotionally tortured through specific patterns of behavior lifetime after lifetime. *Until now!*

Because the 3rd Dimensional world is an experience of loss, fear, and separation, humans naturally create experiences destined to fail. Our intimate experiences are fleeting and marked by emotional highs and lows that denote a false sense of connection. We literally have a relationship with our dreams, ideas, or beliefs about the experiences we are having. That is the essence of a delusion. But this delusion is one that the entire civilization shares. We fall in love only to fall out of love. We have the perfect job, only to be disappointed when it fails to meet our expectations. We live in the most wonderful place, until it isn't so wonderful anymore. Delusional human intimacy is a real 3rd Dimensional experience that promotes discontent, emptiness, and a constant searching for that which is missing.

Soul intimacy is created from a deep sense of purpose and meaning within our connectedness. It is based in the reality of our inherent Oneness and permeates our individual lives in uniquely sacred ways. Our 5th Dimensional relationships are always purposeful. They are never casual, nor do they waste an ounce of our life force on concerns that are significant in the 3rd Dimensional world. Soul intimacy provides evolving human beings with an experience of intimate reverence that facilitates collaboration, equality, and a deep sense of appreciation for the role that is being played, the service being offered, and the loving that is unfolding. In this knowing of all that is involved in 5th Dimensional relationships, we experience a deep sense of satisfaction, joy, and love.

Because 3rd Dimensional relationships are fragile creations in the human mind and heart, they need to be grounded into physical expression to make them "real." Physical exertion is the out-picturing of the internal idea or dream into 3rd Dimensional experience. Thus, sex makes a delusional human intimate relationship physically real. These physical experiences are more 3rd Dimensional energy and offer the dual experience of success or failure, winning or losing, becoming part of or being abandoned, and 3rd Dimensional physical experiences are not only fragile, they end. The concert is over, the competition is completed, a sexual relationship falls apart. Humans are left empty, even after successful moments, looking for ever more physical validation.

Note that 5th Dimensional relationships energetically build upon the connections calling them into being, whether physically, emotionally, mentally, or spiritually. Creativity emerges from these connections and expresses itself through multidimensional sensuality. The electromagnetic energies of unconditional loving and creative collaboration move through the physical cells of the body, allowing the human form to transmit 5th Dimensional frequencies into 3rd

Dimensional physical experiences. This is a continuous experience of life force creatively moving through all your senses. Touch becomes a means of energetic expression rather than physical labor. Sight, sound, hearing, and taste become purposeful venues through which unconditional loving unfolds in specific ways that support the evolution of all involved in the relationship. This is the basis through which energy work, such as Reiki or healing touch, facilitates healing of the 3rd Dimensional body.

3rd Dimensional relationships are self-esteem busters because they rely on external confirmation to determine their validity. Because the relationship is built for a 3rd Dimensional experience of separation and failure, mental insecurity and emotional volatility are necessarily inherent in the process. We seek acknowledgment and praise for whatever we accomplish and tend to feel hurt or disrespected if approval is not provided. The human ego is ever vigilant, scanning for danger to what it considers to be successful. Divorce, getting fired, being thrown off the team or out of the band constitute human failure. Enough failures and your sense of self becomes hurt, then disfigured.

5th Dimensional relationships generate self-esteem. As you become aware of your power to lovingly co-create with another, your respect and appreciation for yourself as well as the other grow. The focus of your attention is internal as you grow in life force and multidimensional awareness, understanding the importance of your relationship and its greater purpose in the world. As a 5th Dimensional collaborator, you show up in relationships already committed to the work at hand and confident of your talents and abilities. You are eager to embrace the unfolding process supporting the others involved and being supported yourself. You experience the opportunity to contribute to the evolution of the world as a gift that you have to give, and for which you will be honored.

3rd Dimensional relationships engage power struggles to promote dominance and submission. In the dualistic plane of the 3rd Dimension, the ego creates dramas that ensnare the heart and enslave the body. War results internally, within families, and among nations. 3rd Dimensional life is already fragile, but without external allegiances, that fragility gives way to a fearful vulnerability that bursts into panic. Whenever an idea, dream, or experience is threatened in the 3rd Dimension, those humans sharing that perspective seek each other out to prove themselves right, just, valid, and significant, regardless of the cost. Human life is expendable if you are not on the same side. And someone else tells you what side you should be on. Whether it be in court, governmental offices, houses of worship, or neighbors' kitchens, human beings look to each other for like-minded support and recognition of worth.

For those experiencing 5th Dimensional relationships, vulnerability builds unconditional loving. Because they are energetically connected to the source of creativity, 5th Dimensional soul-embodied human beings look within for support, direction, and guidance. They trust themselves so that they can show up for each other completely, clearly, and openly. They are collaborators trusting that each is devoted to the highest evolutionary choices available. Open to learning all there is to know and flowing into mutual experiences with respect and appreciation, they honor each other and life itself as it unfolds. They are flexible, creative, ingenious, and filled with wonder as they work together on projects that serve the greater good and contribute to a life of peace. Their experience of vulnerability offers safety as a way of life.

Human beings living 3rd Dimensionally have to be in control of their relationships; otherwise, they will fall apart. Since they are built to break, these fragile relationships must be buttressed by external sources in a recognized pattern of activity that supports their viability. Families literally keep each other alive in many parts of the world. Corporations follow protocols to make profits that keep them in business and their employees working. Governments create policies that support the functioning of their nations according to the resources available on their lands and the productivity of their citizenry. These linear necessities comprise the experience of 3rd Dimensional living and require controlled responses to support this dimensional experience of life.

Fifth Dimensional life is an experience of quantum mechanics while living in a human body. It is the fluid participation of multidimensionally living within the unity of Creation. The concept of Divine timing is helpful in understanding the quantum experience of situations, relationships, and opportunities unfolding at precise moments that change the course of an individual's life, the life of a family, the future of a business, the stability of a nation, the health of a civilization. Creativity is the hallmark by which quantum responses to unfolding experiences occur. Energy is directed to assist and support simultaneously within multiple dimensions so that all engaged are given what is required for them to fulfill themselves in their respective dimensional opportunities.

The human mind cannot comprehend multidimensional mechanics. It is, however, affected by it in the form of guidance, inspiration, and intuition. The most obvious experience of quantum mechanics in 3rd Dimensional living is grace.

Because 3rd Dimensional relationships are not meant to last, they will inevitably incur multiple experiences of dying. Death, the ultimate form of separation, happens slowly in the loss of hopes and dreams, or quickly as in being fired from a job or the accidental death of a loved one. Whether fast or slow, an irreconcilable experience of loss creates a spiritual crisis. However, in the earthly experience, death began to reinforce the disintegration of the heart of humanity and furthered its descent into the ego of physicality. Lost in the desire to prolong life at all costs, the purpose of living was lost to the experience of living. Without a compass by which to understand life, humanity created its own spiral of deathly discontent, almost annihilating itself.

Because 5th Dimensional relationships consciously exist within the unity of Creation, connection is already a lived experience. As purpose guides relationships to fulfillment and collaboration supports multidimensional celebration, life is honored in every phase of its existence. Completion is valued and honored. It is not experienced as death. Evolution is recognized as the source of continuity within and between dimensions. Instead of mourning the loss of connection with a loved one, another greater level of relationship emerges. However, this level of contact is only possible from the 5th Dimensional perspective in and through which you continue to meet each other. The common description of Heaven as a place of peace, safety, love, and beauty is a 3rd Dimensional expression of 5th Dimensional living. It has been placed as otherworldly because, up until now, you had to die to experience it. This is no longer the case.

5th Dimensional relationships energetically build upon the connections calling them into being physically, emotionally, mentally, and spiritually. Creativity emerges from these connections and expresses itself through multidimensional sensuality. The electromagnetic energies of unconditional loving and creative collaboration move through the physical cells of the body, allowing the human form to transmit 5th Dimensional frequencies into 3rd Dimensional physical experiences. This is a continuous experience of life force creatively moving through all your senses. Touch becomes a means of energetic expression rather than physical labor. Sight, sound, hearing, and taste become purposeful venues through which unconditional loving unfolds in specific ways.

5th Dimensional *relationships are no longer a dream on Earth.* They are realities that we make each day by choosing higher-dimensional responses to 3rd Dimensional experiences. We are an evolving species whose intimate relationships chart the course for the future of a soul-embodied humanity. Developing your personal 5th Dimensional relationships is the perfect place to start experiencing the reality of 5th Dimensional, unconditionally loving joy. As you do, you pioneer the way for others to grow into the courage and grace you are lovingly offering to the world right now.

The 5D relationship gives each other a great deal of love, respect, and support. We are not dependent on each other's love to feel good about ourselves, or to feel valuable and important. The love we receive from others is a bonus, an overflow that is much appreciated and valued, but is not needed at the core of our being because we are able to provide the love we need from within ourselves. There is, therefore, no emotional demand that those we're in relationship with give us the love we need to feel good about ourselves.

A CHANNELED UNDERSTANDING OF THE 5TH DIMENSIONAL CONSCIOUSNESS

As we move from the 3rd Dimension, it can feel heavy and difficult, especially during this time in history. When you experience a transformation, you may feel sad, depressed, as if your life situations are worsening. We are undergoing a mass movement into the 5th Dimension, and that is where the magic and Miracles happen.

There is an unknown aspect of this transition that you know you cannot control. It can feel like mourning as you let go and surrender to God's will. Personal empowerment amid this uncomfortable change is in knowing a higher power will flow through you. **One way it will demonstrate itself is through your gifts that you feel compelled to share with the world. You begin to feel confident, strengthened, with an interest in self-care and a feeling of personal possibility.**

There may still be moments of brief sadness as you let go of the 3rd Dimension, but they will be less intense. In this zone, you'll begin to feel as if you're on a mission, there is something that you must do, that must pass through you as a Divine vessel.

Those with 5th Dimensional consciousness will move and migrate toward each other. Some will move back and forth between the dimensions while others will anchor the 5th Dimension. This is called bouncing back and forth from one Dimension to another. You will also need to be spiritually understanding that you may still have moments when you feel sad, concerned, or even afraid. However, as your consciousness rises, you will come to know that these feelings are not you. They are momentary experiences of feelings that will pass.

You now understand that you will not be deterred from adhering to the higher energy that now pulls you toward a higher vision. Even though our lives have shifted, my Guides want us to honor the Omnipresent even more by creating a pure loving connection and faith. The more we stop the fear and put love into our hearts and serve others, the more we can positively shift the energy. The old paradigm is over, and this is okay. We are all right, and the Divine will see us through this challenge.

There may be individuals who are still not comfortable with these higher energies. These individuals may choose to remain in the 3rd Dimension. It is their free will. However, their life experience will not be as easy. My Guides tell me the way we can evolve in society is through DNA activation. Eventually, the body adjusts, and it will no longer experience the symptoms as it did in the past.

Even though messages are specific to each person, in my workshops and online classes, I often hold large group meditations and activations. This can be done if we are all focused on a singular global message like world peace, compassion, and cohesion. I often will use a camera focused directly on my eyes that allows everyone in the group to focus on them. My Guides now tell me I also have the ability to activate healings through the hands. They want me to teach people how to be prayer healers through their hands. With God, all things are possible.

If we can surrender over and just be in this beautiful higher Dimension, we can be healed. Our Guides want us to have faith in ourselves and our gifts and to be the authentic loving beings that we are. They want us to be fearless and loving and know that we are powerful souls.

THE DIVINE FEMININE WITHIN US

Divine feminine energy is comprised of the following Angelic qualities—unconditional love, understanding, compassion, nurturing, and helpfulness to others. It includes tenderness, gentleness, kindness, and all the other Divine feelings you might relate to unconditional love—the greatest of all God's Divine cosmic powers. The unconditional love within Divine feminine energy has a powerful magnetic quality. At its highest level of 5th Dimensional conscious Oneness with God, unconditional love has the power to heal, to harmonize, and to create Miracles just as Jesus did so long ago.

The Divine feminine energy is here now more than ever, making its way in passive nature. It is this passivity, this peace, love (experienced by the stilling of the ego-influenced, finite human brain-mind) that opens the heart's spiritual door to the soul and permits the human self to receive—intuitively—Divine guidance and information from the Divine mind and loving heart of his or her very own Divine eternal soul and God Within.

"Be still and know I Am God," which means be still in your human brain-mind (as in meditation) and begin to know, to remember, to feel, and to realize for yourself the Divine energies, qualities, and attributes of the Spark of Goddessness in YOU. There are powerful prayers for this in the next section of the book.

And now it's time to dive into the beauty of the 5th Dimension through powerful practices!

5TH DIMENSION SOUL:
PRACTICES FOR HEALING

The following chapters contain life-transforming prayers, affirmations, and more. Use them to empower your life, to strengthen your body and mind, and to lift your spiritual awareness to the 5th Dimension. It is in the 5th Dimension that healing can take place quickly. It is also in the 5th Dimension that we can thrive and live authentically in our Divine nature.

There is also a chapter about chakras and how to use chakras the 5th Dimension way. As we learn in the 5th Dimension, everything is energy, including our bodies, so learning about chakra energy, and how to direct it with focus, can bring powerful change to your life.

People ask me if they have to attend a class or have a private session with me to experience the 5th Dimension. I let them know that **the 5th Dimension is available to everyone, all the time. The techniques, prayers, affirmations, and practices in this book are ways that people can begin to develop the practice of entering the 5th Dimension in their own lives.**

Read through these chapters, and then come back and use the material over and over throughout your life.

PRAYERS:

AFFIRMATIONS:

EXERCISES:

CHAKRA:

4

5TH DIMENSION PRAYERS AND AFFIRMATIONS

Prayers and affirmations are ways we can connect directly with God. In 5th Dimension language, that means **we can use prayers and affirmations to lift our vibration up from a 3D experience to a 5D experience.** You can read them quietly, or you can read them aloud. Either way, as you read them, breathe deeply, keep focused on the words, and then feel how the words uplift you. Repeat them as often as you need to feel uplifted.

PRAYERS:
MODERN-DAY MOTHER MARY PRAYER

The following healing prayer brings in a relationship with the feminine Divine. Embracing both our masculine and feminine energies allows each of us to be a receptive force for good and create much-needed balance in today's world. This prayer can be used at any time for any purpose.

We honor our beautiful Divine Mother Mary!

I honor the feminine Divine in you
in this everyday world
all forms of the Divine
shifting the energy to love
I honor the feminine
Divine energy in myself as well
to serve others, I serve you

Freely balancing the masculine energy
choosing to not cling to any energy
that binds me
or does not serve me
I rinse off the shame

My eyes shine
my heart is worth the gold of God's love

I live in my truth
I live in my feminine strength

I can speak freely now
I can speak strongly about who I am
to you and for you

In that I am free
I am the Feminine Divine
I carry all my wounds
I fill my cup up with holy water
and my right hand swears to always
be a modern-day Mother Mary
in this everyday world
shifting the energy to Love.

I AM LIGHT—A CHANNELED PRAYER

When I pray to God, it's always with an open heart. I thank God and never ask or want.

You can even pray to Mary and Jesus and all the saints and the Angelic realm.

Acknowledge God's greatness. If you have faith in God, you believe in the Divine Creator of the world and all life on Earth, the Divine will Believe in you and come to your side.

This is my heartfelt prayer to God.

Dear beloved Holy One
I honor your loving presence
in my life
I thank you so much
for everything
in my life
and all that you provide
for me
and my friends
and family

Despite the burdens
that lie on my shoulders
in this 3rd Dimension world
such as financial hardship
sickness
or shadowing depression
I am
turning it all over to you

fully
and saying
I am love
I am light
I believe in Miracles
and that my mind,
body,
and conscious Spirit
can be healed
lifted by your love
and that true abundance
can happen

I am fully connected
to be aided in my needs
or in the needs of others
when I ask fully
with an open heart
to assist my loved one

I know the Angels
are also healing me
and guiding my healing

Dear Holy Spirit
I am your humble servant
I am your child
I believe in Christ
I'm so thankful
you love me so faithfully

and keep me safe
in the highest Dimension
of pure grace

I am healed
I am yours
I am light.

AWAKEN ME, O FEMININE DIVINE

Please read the poem below as you bring in your Divine Feminine energy and as you open your heart chakra. This is a channeled message to enhance the Divine Feminine and Divine Masculine to balance the blessed energy in your body. It can be recited out loud or quietly to yourself.

Awaken within me,
O Feminine Divine!

Bring forth
the flame
of your knowledge
of all things
material
and spiritual

Awaken within me,
O Feminine Divine!

Bring forth
the blessed waters
of your wisdom
in all things
material
and spiritual

Bring forth
your softness

Bring forth
your clarity

Bring forth
your wisdom

Bring forth
the best in me

Awaken me,
O Feminine Divine
to your Divine self

Awaken me,
O Feminine Divine
to yourself in me

Awaken me,
O Feminine Divine
to myself

Awaken me,
O Feminine Divine
to myself in me

Awaken me,
O Feminine Divine
from my world of illusions

Awaken me,
O Feminine Divine
to your Divine truth

Awaken me,
O Feminine Divine
from my world of illusions

Awaken me
O Feminine Divine
to the truth in you

I become myself
as I awaken
within you

I become myself
as you awaken
within me

I become myself
as I awaken
within you

I become myself
as you awaken
within me

Blossom within me,
O Feminine Divine

bloom brightly
your knowledge
of all things
material
and spiritual

Bloom within me,
O Feminine Divine
the bountiful
and beautiful
blossoms
of your wisdom
in all things
material
and spiritual

Amen.

THE MIRACULOUS HEALING PRAYER

This powerful prayer can be used for any medical condition or challenge, whether physical, mental, or emotional. If you or a loved one confronts immune suppression, cancer, heart disease, diabetes, hormone imbalance, thyroid issues, infections, mental despair, or any other condition not mentioned here, this prayer, when prayed with a sincere heart, can bring healing benefits or improvement.

When we call on the miraculous power of the Holy Spirit, the quantum field can not only expand the rhythm of your flow, but you can be heard and instantly healed. My belief is that the prayers that enable you to speak and express your voice and needs to Christ Consciousness work best when you speak and live as though your prayers have already been answered.

> *I remove all fear and doubt from my heart by the power of the Holy Spirit.*
> *May You know, my Lord, that I glorify You*
> *I pray that You know that my heart is sincere*
> *I pray to You that You comfort me in my suffering*
> *I pray that You lend me skills in my hands like the hands of the Healer, that You are to heal me, to lend me strength to heal myself and give me the power and grace to accept my healing right now.*
> *I deserve to be healed! I am humble. I am not afraid. I put my whole trust in You. I love You.*
> *I know by the power of the love of Christ Consciousness and Jesus and all my highest Guides and the Angelic Realm*

that this [say your condition] and whatever negative energy affects me, I now breathe out of my body. It no longer resides in my energy field or my mind, or my body, or my Spirit. All illness, all negativity, is gone. I am a believer. You are my Healer right now, and You have HEALED me.

I am so grateful to have my breath. I breathe love, and I am flowing in this amazing higher quantum 5th Dimension. I am healed.

I know You have saved me. I know You are restoring my health through my thoughts and through my body right now. I know that You hear me right now. I believe and I know through the grace of Christ Consciousness I feel good and loved by You. I have no fear, only love and light. I feel amazing. My physical being is healed.

El Shaddai and the power of God reside in me, and I glorify You and I am glorified in You!

Amen.

THE 5TH DIMENSIONAL MIRACLE PRAYER

I am fully, freely, and willingly accepting today the Awakening of the 5th Dimension.

I know and trust that by fully being in the 5th Dimension, I will witness Miracles today.

My heart is open and ready to receive the love and intimacy of God Consciousness.

When fully trusting God in the 5th Dimension, I can hear and feel and have a shift, and everything in my life is easy and abundant.

Through the Divine, my gifts are fully awakened today in the 5th Dimension.

I am healed in the 5th Dimension. I feel amazing in the 5th Dimension.

I love being in the 5th Dimension.

I feel peace, love, and joy in the 5th Dimension.

I am trusting that the negative 3rd Dimensional mind chatter is quickly overcome by the 5th Dimension.

My mind is automatically focused on the present moment with no effort required.

My mind is simply a state of being.

I automatically live in the 5th Dimension.

My heart is open in the 5th Dimension.

I am a child of God.

THE MAGICAL 5TH DIMENSIONAL PEACE PRAYER

*I love being in the magical
5th Dimensional frequency
of love
and peace
where all is pure,
existence is nonjudgmental,
and awareness is beyond
all time,
all space,
and all place*

*In the magical 5th Dimension,
humans can
do all,
be all,
and thereby find
miraculous healing*

*the love of the Omnipresent
is centered on all civilizations
to have one underlying focus
of peace and service*

*love is simple and easy
in the 5th Dimension,
moving our world*

into
a gigantic
organic
global field
where healing is easy and fast

Because we are dimensional beings,
our minds want to live in this existence
where the Omnipresent exists
gentle, safe, pure, and respectful
with the flow of Spirit
guiding us to be strong
building daily intimacy with God Divine.

Therefore, I am healed.

THE 5TH DIMENSION PRAYER FOR FORGIVENESS

This prayer can be used to forgive others or to forgive yourself. Use this often; never hold on to negative energy. Forgiveness doesn't mean agreement; forgiveness is a way for you to let go of energy that holds you down, and it allows you to move forward.

Dear Holy Spirit,
please help me to remember
the power of forgiveness,
and please help me to extend
forgiveness to [say person's name]
and to myself.
I know what it means to forgive,
and I know all the things
for which You have forgiven me.
Despite my feelings
about [person's name],
please help me
to remember that
You love [person's name]
and You care about their well-being.
Please help me
to find love in my heart
and to move past
what was said and done.
Please help me
to forgive [person's name]
and to move past this hurt,

leaving it in the 3rd Dimension.
I pray to all the saints
and Angels
and Christ light.
I pray for Your comfort
and assistance
And I thank You,
because I am
in the 5th Dimension.
Amen.

THE 5TH DIMENSION PRAYER OF GRATITUDE

Being in a state of gratitude is a powerful way to experience the 5th Dimension. The 5th Dimension experience is a way to be fully content, fully aware, and fully open to Spirit. Gratitude is the doorway to a different way of seeing your life.

Oh Jesus, Angels,
and all the prophets,
I truly know I can only show you
so much gratitude
for my life and blessings
by being your humble servant
and doing as I am told.

Thank you for guiding me
to help humanity and all living creatures
Give me the attitude
of thankful daily gratitude
I know that your truth
dwells in a thankful heart.
I know that giving without wanting
anything in return
brings my life to its fullest
and has a universal effect
of Ascension.
I live in trust,
I live in the present moment
of being at peace.
Amen.

THE 5TH DIMENSION BLESSING PRAYER FOR MEALS AND FOOD THROUGH THE HOLY SPIRIT

Being in a state of gratitude extends to what we put inside our bodies. Use this prayer—or one that you create—to use your mealtimes as ways to remember your 5th Dimension reality.

Thank you, God,
for Your presence
with us.
Bless this food for our bodies,
so that we may be
strong to serve,
gracious in giving,
and overflowing with love.
Thank You, God,
for this nourishment,
for the warmth of the sun,
for the refreshment of pure water,
for the Miracle of the harvest,
and for sacred love,
which energizes taste
and blesses this food.
Thank You, God,
for giving us
Your Divine holy loving energy
through our food.
Thank You, God.

THE 5TH DIMENSION PRAYER OF PROTECTION

It can seem that in the 3rd Dimension world, everyone and everything is trying to scare us. The news knows that reporting what frightens us will keep us tuned in . . . but it also means that we are tuned in to the energy of fear. Our family and friends can sometimes impose their fear onto us. But in the 5th Dimension, we rise above fear and enter into the grounded state of being of love. This doesn't mean we ignore the world around us; rather, it means that we are now effective beings of Light in the world. We are in our power.

I am not afraid
I am in the 5th Dimension
and the Holy Spirit
is completely protecting me.
I am a multidimensional being
making a clear choice to experience prayer
in this Dimension.
The 5th Dimension
combats against dark energy!
I am love and I am light
and all my fears are released.
The perfect love
of the Christ Consciousness
is here.
I am love,
and joy,
and I have no fear.
Amen.

THE 5TH DIMENSION MORNING HEALING PRAYER

Start your day with this prayer, so that you begin each day in the highest energy.

Good morning, Creator,
Good morning, Angels.
Please stay with me,
today and every day,
wherever I go.
Please give me strength,
today and every day,
whatever I do.
Let me have no danger,
today and every day,
whatever I face.
Today and every day,
let no task
overcome me.
Today and every day,
let no trial
overcome my heart.
Today and every day,
I am in the 5th Dimension!
My consciousness
is strong,
my energy
and my mind
are healthy!
I shall have courage,

*whatever my day
shall bring.
My protection shield
is made of Christ light!
I know my Divine mission.
I am in the 5th Dimension!
Amen.*

THE 5TH DIMENSION EVENING HEALING PRAYER

Say this prayer just before sleeping, so that you end each day in that 5th Dimension energy.

Dear God,
thank You for another day of life.
I am thankful for my friends
and family and for all
Your beautiful creations.
I love You.
Thank You for my life.
Thank You for all
Your positive energy
overflowing and abundant.
I am overjoyed
to be experiencing
the 5th Dimensional energy
in my daily life.
Thank You for my health.
I have unconditional love
and compassion for all.
Amen.

AFFIRMATIONS:
WE ARE MULTIDIMENSIONAL BEINGS

I live in a multidimensional world
with many multidimensional beings.

Love is multidimensional
I view love from every angle

I choose to have
the highest
God awareness.
I don't suffer
I am healed

I am a beautiful
multidimensional
being

My soul loves living
in a multidimensional world
I am
immortal,
infinite
and divine
I don't suffer
I am healed.

I AM HEALED

Love is God
and God is love
every cell in my body
is white light
I am leaving behind
3rd Dimensional worry, pain, and fear
I am strong
and loved
in the magical Dimension
of cosmic light
I am in love
with the 5th Dimensional cosmic consciousness.
I feel so amazing and safe.
I am love.
I am light.
This is magical.
I am joy.
And I am healed.
This is magical.
I am joy.
And I am healed.

5TH DIMENSION DNA AWAKENING

My eyes
have been awakened
to the 12th Dimensional blueprint
of my DNA.

My DNA strands
have been activated
in the 5th Dimension.

My DNA strands are youthful and strong!

I am powerful
I speak clearly
I see clearly
I am creative
I am grounded
I am fearless

I am in a truthful state of reality
of Divine sovereign consciousness.
The Universe is at peace.
I am at peace.

5D STARSEED

I am born a Starseed born in a 3rd Dimensional body
I am a Starseed, an Angelic light being
I am here on this earth plane

I was sent here to complete a mission
My purpose is to help humanity in some way
I am a Starseed to assist the earth and humanity with the
*   Ascension process*

The Ascension involves raising the energy to a higher
*   vibrational frequency*
To shift the consciousness into a heart-based conscious Universe
We are Starseeds, the 11:11 triggers an Awakening of the
*   Starseeds as we move humanity forward*

I am born a Starseed born in a 3rd Dimensional body
I am a Starseed, an Angelic light being
I am here on this earth plane

I walk my path to the Awakening
As many other Starseeds join together and open up their hearts
*   to the Divine Light mission*
We can all save the Universe.

ANGELS IN THE 5TH DIMENSION

I'm in the 5th Dimension
I love being in the 5th Dimension
I have left the 3rd Dimensional challenges and difficulties
*   behind*
I'm accepting my Archangels and the changes I will face in the
*   5th Dimension with grace*

I am ready for the love, peace, and abundance
that I deserve
In all of the spiritual guidance of the Holy Divine in the 5th
*   Dimension, I have more access through my Spirit Guides*
My Angels are Awakening my abilities more every day and are
*   readily and easily accessible in the 5th Dimension*

I feel safe in the Angelic realm
I know I am love and I am light
I know that time is easier in the 5th Dimension
I know I am more intimate with the Divine God in the 5th
*   Dimension*
My thoughts are more focused on the positive

I have more energy
I have more access to my Spirit Guides and Angels, and my
*   abilities are heightened in the 5th Dimension*

I can breathe easily
I've been awakened from birth

I'm in the 5th Dimension
I am healed in the 5th Dimension
I love being in the 5th Dimension
I'm empathetic to people and circumstances
My core heart is opened and caring

I am protected by the Holy One, God, and all my Angels that
    are truly the messengers
I am relaxed
I let go
I surrender
I remember this is a journey
I am in the Dimension of love and joy
I am in the Awakening and I am in the 5th Dimension

I know my Angels love me
I feel them more every day
I feel their support in this journey as I move forward in this
    learning and serving in the 5th Dimensional love.

AWAKENED ANGELS

*My real self knows my awakened Angel and the intention for
me being here.*

*It is time to step into my true consciousness or higher knowing
and set my wings free.*

*I speak in harmony with my Angelic light codes through the
guidance and the awakened ones.*

*My body is a stream of light, an Angelic wisdom in step of pure
white love here to be visible to those who wish to see me.*

*I am an awakened Angel, a healing light force helping to
empower you.*

Take you on a journey through a parallel Universe.

The experience is the brilliance in you and the awakened Angels.

The empowered steps for you take to open your eyes.

My real self knows my awakened Angel is real and here for me.

Is now and true I am a host for this reality and to be set free.

My Angel wings to be free.

*I can sing and see above the mountains and look out farther
than the sea.*

I know my Angels are always with me.

I am Awakened, I am the Awakened one.

5TH DIMENSION EXERCISES

The following are several powerful exercises to align your soul, body, and mind to the 5th Dimension. Read through each exercise fully before beginning, so you understand each exercise completely. In general, it's a good idea to find a quiet place to do these exercises, so you can fully focus and not be interrupted. However, you can, of course, use them anywhere needed, provided you aren't driving or operating machinery or need to focus on something else.

Each of these exercises will help bring you into the 5th Dimension and help to change your energy, your awareness, and your life.

AWAKENING THE SUPER CONSCIOUSNESS IN OUR BREATH

Go to a place where you can be comfortable and not interrupted. Take a breath, clear your mind, become present. When you're ready, start with step 1.

> Step 1: Sitting upright, slowly inhale through your nose. Slowly exhale through your mouth, getting all the oxygen out of your lungs . . .
>
> Step 2: Slowly inhale deeply through your nose to the count of four . . .
>
> Step 3: Hold your breath for a count of four . . .
>
> Step 4: Exhale again to the count of four . . .
>
> Step 5: Hold your breath again for a count of four, and repeat these steps.

I love to guide my clients to imagine your crown chakra opening, like a blossom opening to the sun. Breathe in the bright white-golden light from the cosmic central sun. Use your in-breath to direct the light through your brain, through every chakra, down to your root chakra.

Hold your breath for a moment, use the root lock (contract your pelvic muscle) while you breathe out, slowly and gently, observing the light flowing up from your root chakra through your spine and upward to your crown chakra. Release the root chakra and relax.

Note: You'll learn more about chakras in the next chapter.

5TH DIMENSION THIRD EYE PINEAL GLAND MEDITATION EXERCISE: AWAKENING INTO THE 5TH DIMENSION

The purpose of this meditation is to pull the mind out of the body so as to draw the energy of the body's first five energy centers (physical, vital, mental, super mental, and bliss) back up to the brain.

The third eye is our greatest gift to connect us to source and remind us of a Universe much more mystical than that which we perceive with our physical senses. The third eye is the spiritual part of us that "sees" through a higher energy. It's through the Awakening of the third eye and its corresponding pineal gland that we're able to attain supernatural gifts of telepathy, psychic vision, and an intimate connection with God. Our purpose is to awaken our crown chakra to empower the super consciousness. This is the highest form of enlightenment. The light is then fully awakened and fully free within your soul purpose.

Here are some of the signs your third eye is opening:

- A dull sensation of pressure between the eyebrows . . .
- Increased foresight . . .
- Prone to light sensitivity . . .
- A feeling of gradual and continual change . . .
- Increased headaches.

When you do the twenty-minute pineal gland meditation to induce the mystical moment, sit up longer than you normally would in a meditation. This is important because if you sit up past the point where your body wants to lie down, your body is going to surrender more deeply to your Guides and your Angels. It's in this state of relaxation and satisfaction when the door to the mystical opens. This is essential because if you want to operate in that realm between wakefulness and sleep, your body has to *feel* like it's asleep, while at the same time your mind has to be awake. As you pass through that little doorway, through that portal, it causes you to again enter another world. You become very conscious in your subconscious mind.

It's also important to add here that if you really want to have a great mystical experience, do your meditation somewhere other than your bed so you're not as likely to immediately fall asleep. When you do lie down, it helps if you put a pillow or a bolster under your knees so that you feel relaxed and comfortable, but it doesn't *feel* like you are in bed.

The purpose of any meditation is to connect to your breath and pull your mind out of the body so as to draw the energy of the body's first three energy centers (crown chakra, root chakra, and heart chakra) back up to the brain. The breath comes in a slow, steady inhalation as you contract your abdominal muscles at the same time. Meanwhile, follow your breath all the way to the pineal gland, located in the third cerebral ventricle of the brain. The pineal gland is commonly known as the Third Eye, located deep in the center of the brain. When your awareness reaches your sixth chakra (third eye), hold your breath and further squeeze those intrinsic muscles again.

As you push cerebral spinal fluid up against the crystals of the pineal gland, which happens while doing this breath exercise, it activates latent systems that cause the pineal gland (the gland that's responsible for the transcendental experience) to become electrically stimulated. This electrical current causes the crystals in the pineal gland to magically awaken. The pineal gland then transduces the frequencies into profound light (an Awakening).

As we breathe with eyes closed, enhancing the mind and the body and back into the brain, the brain can go into heightened brain wave states. This is beyond the 5th Dimension and higher, and activates the God Consciousness, connecting you to your Divine power, the light of God.

Keeping the Rhythm of the 5th Dimension Breath

As you do this exercise, it will also require you to change the beliefs you're tied to, such as you'll be too tired during the day and/or that you'll be in a bad mood as a result of not having enough energy. It's important to do five to ten minutes a day of breathing exercises.

Once the door to the super consciousness (the power of the Miracle mind) opens to you, because you have been knocking on the door every day, you will say what every person says when their moment comes: it will open your third eye.

You will be revealed to yourself, and you will never be the same person again. You will finally understand that the only way to get to the super you (super you and super me are the amplified superheroes within each of us) is to leave behind everything known to you—so much so that you will want to get beyond your known self every day and open up to the real possibility of a fearless life, which is in the 5th Dimension.

To be selfless in serving humanity is to lose yourself to the unknown every day. Once you know the formula of how to get there, this new way of learning the technique of getting into this Dimension is easy and fun and super cool. Super consciousness health is a breath formula that will awaken your life.

5TH DIMENSION DREAM JOURNAL EXERCISE

A dream diary or dream journal can help you reduce stress, inspire your creativity, and connect you to your deeper subconscious. It provides an ongoing record to help you re-member dreams so you can analyze them later.

Every now and then, set an alarm to wake up in the middle of your meditation, to write down your dreams in a journal—or at least the last thing you remembered from your dreams. If you can recall the dream, you are literally learn-ing how to stay conscious in the subconscious realm. Once you do that, the next step is to review the dream.

As you get good at it, the dream becomes animate again, and now you're back in the dream world consciously. When you're conscious in your dream, this is when lucid dreaming starts to occur (the act of being aware that you are dreaming, while doing it, gives you more control over the dream, hence the term *lucid dreaming*).

5TH DIMENSION MOTHER MARY ENERGY: A HIGH-VIBRATION FIELD EXERCISE

While doing a hands-on healing, I repeat the Mother Mary prayer: "Hail Mary, full of grace, the Lord is with thee. Blessed art thou among women, and blessed is the fruit of thy womb, Jesus. Holy Mary, Mother of God, pray for us sinners, now and at the hour of our death. Amen."

Mother Mary helps us to get a sense of God's action and presence in the world and connects us to our feminine Divine energy. This channeled exercise is very beneficial in putting harmony together with our masculine and feminine light body.

Now I'm going to teach you how to do this. First, rub your hands together vigorously for several seconds to invoke the Divine within you. As the Holy Divine is honoring YOU, you are Honoring the Holy Divine, God. The next step is rubbing your palms together again and then placing your hands around your neck; perhaps apply some rose oil before rubbing, and breathe again three times, saying a prayer such as "I accept the Holy Spirit, and through accepting the Holy Spirit, I am healed." Or use any prayer you feel in your heart. Then rub your hands together again a third time and again place your hands on your neck, and then on any part of your body in need of healing.

Say, "I release all the negative energy out of my body, out of the room, and out of the Universe NOW! Amen."

Repeat this mantra at least twice a day with some soothing beautiful background music on. This activates the serotonin in your brain, which is connected to the deeper Holy

Divine mother love and the 5th Dimensional energy. You repeat out loud at the end, "I am Awakening to this healing energy in the 5th Dimension. My whole body is shifted into this loving Dimension, every cell is healed, all the DNA in my body is being transformed by Spirit communicating out loud and being healed. Namaste." The crown chakra is awakened and blessed.

It is a constant honoring of the healing that is going on. As you continue saying a blessed mantra or prayer, you are invoking it in the body. You experience being in your body with your breath. You breathe in life. The last step is to check the lymph glands, to rub your hands together and place them alongside your throat.

Remember that a high-vibration field shields you from negative energies. It can keep your immune system strong, build a strong relationship with the Divine feminine loving Mother healing energy, and give you a daily alignment with Spirit.

You will have learned how to be in the God Frequency.

12TH DIMENSION SHIELD BUBBLE OF PROTECTION

(This involves creating an energetic safety shield in a multidimensional Universe.)

This powerful shielding and grounding exercise can be used wherever you need it, including anytime you feel worry or anxiety.

The 12th Dimension is being completely one with God. You can draw upon the 12D like a shield to protect yourself here in the 3D. Once a person is attuned and working with the 12D Shield daily, the Lightbody (the energetic counterpart of the physical body) becomes aligned to the 12th Dimension. At a certain level of proficiency, one can utilize the 12D Shield as a transit gate vortex, or a shadow gate. This is a vortex set up specifically to clear lower-vibration energies (lost human souls that didn't transcend to the light), entities, and negativity from the space one commands within the 12D Shield. This means one is stating an intention to clear out lower 3rd Dimensional frequencies, misplaced entities (lost human souls), or negative energies that accumulate in a room, space, or group aura field through having exposure to higher frequencies.

When one is choosing to consent to the God Frequency, you're aligning with the Law of One (the infinite Creator). You are therefore entering into the 12D Energy Shield. When entering a space, you have the ability to command the field to be cleared of lower frequencies.

When entering into your field of space and time, you're ordering lower frequencies—misplaced energies and negative entities that have entered into a room, space, or field—to clear out. Examples: airport terminals, grocery stores, locations with lots of electromagnetic activity.

To replace these lower energies, you have placed yourself within a sealed 12D bubble of higher frequencies. This is a self-protection seal of God Frequency with a transtate gate vortex within a Merkaba (a sacred geometry symbol, like a star around your body; the vortex is a natural hypnotic state).

This can be a daily exercise. Once you learn this technique, this activation will be easy and simple. The Spirit wants you to learn this so you can easily access the 5th Dimension. The Spirit wants you to have less anxiety and more protection living in the 3rd Dimensional world. You can surround yourself with the 12D Bubble during daily activities, or while sitting or lying down in daily meditations.

Entering the 12D Shield

Breathe and see yourself deep inside a white cloud of light floating across the sky.

As you imagine beautiful eagles flying above you, take deep breaths, inhaling and exhaling, keeping your eyes shut and both your hands out at your sides.

Raise your hands above you, then bring your hands onto your head, over your crown chakra (the area above the top of your head), and trace the shape of a shield all the way around your body.

Place a silver 12th Dimensional Shield Bubble (a cosmic safety shield to strengthen your aura) around your entire body.

Bring your hands over your heart chakra (the middle of your chest).

Say out loud, or to yourself:

I am love.
I am light.
I am safe.

As your eyes are closed within the 12th Dimensional vortex, go back to your deep breathing.

Envision in your heart chakra a place you feel safe, such as floating across the sky, or feeling the ocean breeze while inside this beautiful silver bubble of self-protection. It can be a beach or a cabin in the woods or a real place such as a room in your home.

Imagine a beautiful golden rope, glowing and light. Now with your hands, take this golden rope and tie a bow at the end of your feet, sealing the bubble.

Continue to focus on the Shield Bubble, keeping all negative emotions from affecting you.

Envision the bow wrapped around the end of the seal at the bottom of your feet.

In the center of your 12th Dimensional Shield Bubble, envision a golden ball with a golden rope (the same rope as earlier) going from the solar plexus up to the energy of God the Divine.

Push out the unwanted negative energy from your body, out of the room, out of the Universe, centering your body into a beautiful energy field with the Divine.

Try to focus this energy for at least five minutes in this bubble of self-protection.

Coming Out of the 12D Shield

When coming out of the Shield, slowly take three deep breaths.

You should feel relaxed when you emerge, like your possibilities are endless. The more you practice this powerful exercise, which lasts from twenty to thirty minutes, the more you can become connected to the 5th Dimension.

5TH DIMENSION FORGIVENESS MANTRA

(This technique can be done on your own after watching one of my instructional videos.)

Take both of your hands and place them over your neck and take a breath. Think of a person who has harmed you in the 3rd Dimension and say, "I forgive anyone who has hurt me." (Or you may say a specific person's name.) "And please forgive me. The only thing between me and you is the energy of God."

Take a deep breath, inhale, and exhale. Then let it out of your throat chakra. Repeat this process three times.

Next, place your hands around your throat, sweeping away the negative energy and saying out loud, "I release any negative energy out of my body, out of the room, and out of the Universe now!"

Let's say your issue is with your mother. Say: "I forgive my mother, who has harmed me. Please forgive my mother. Please forgive me." Then let out a large vocal clearing from your throat and say, "The only energy between me and my mother is the energy of God. Amen."

This is a profound clearing mantra.

THE NEW 5TH DIMENSION WAY OF HEALING

When you go inward during prayer or meditation and with music, your energy field is more alive, you're no longer dominated by your thoughts, and you can enter a healing vibration state of love and inner harmony.

The Dimension of God Energy can be brought into your body to diminish stress and strengthen your immune system. I teach people to do this in meditation, using mantras, meaningful chants or sound, or a prayer, to channel and call in the Guides. The Guides will come and assist you in this process. Calling in the Holy Divine in the 5th Dimension is the key to these exercises and building a solid intimacy every day to remain healed. This not only keeps you grounded but centered, focused, and goal oriented in all your life's purposes. Your mind is not on the material world. The 5D is focused on love and the supernatural magic, and in that realm, anything is possible.

What I describe here can be done in group settings or even on Skype webinars by putting your hands up on the computer screen. What I do in public is to say, "We are releasing any negative energy out of our bodies, out of the room, out of the Universe, NOW!" Say that three or four times while doing deep breaths, in and out.

We also chant the Hail Mary, calling in the feminine Divine. We chant Om, we do strong inner peace mantras. You could just say a simple prayer from your childhood, or a sacred prayer used by your family.

It's important you are strongly motivated about the negative energy leaving your body, breathing the negative energy out, telling it to leave, and you are confirming the Holy Spirit with a prayer into the body, asking the energy of the Divine to enter you. This process goes on for fifteen to thirty minutes. As you repeat your mantra or prayer, your thoughts will become loving, kind, peaceful, and holy. That is what the Holy Spirit is—loving, kind, peaceful, and good. This is the energy vibration your body needs to heal itself. When you are feeling worry or fear, you are not in sync with the Divine, so tell the negative energy to leave your body, to go out of the room, out of the Universe, NOW!

If there is an area of your body that is unwell, you can awaken the area by invoking the Spirit through your palms, rubbing your hands together, and placing them on the unwell area. You vocally breathe out the negative energy with an exhalation of breath as you tell the negative energy to leave. This empowers your throat chakra and your throat to release the negative energy through your mouth. Do it again three more times, each time further releasing the energy.

Rubbing your hands together vigorously invokes the Divine within you, as the Holy Divine is honoring YOU. You are Honoring the Holy Divine, God. The next step is rubbing your palms together again and then placing your hands around your neck, perhaps with some rose oil, and breathing again three times, saying a prayer such as "I accept the Holy Spirit, and through acceptance of the Holy Spirit, I am healed." Or use any prayer you feel in your heart. Then rub your hands together again and place them on your neck and then on any part of your body that needs healing.

Say to yourself out loud, "I release all the negative energy out of my body, out of the room, and out of the Universe NOW! Amen."

Repeat this mantra at least three to five times, preferably with some beautiful soothing background music on. This activates the serotonin in your brain, which is connected to the deeper Holy Divine Mother love, as well as the 5th Dimensional energy. You repeat out loud, "I am Awakening to this healing energy in the 5th Dimension. My whole body is shifted into this loving Dimension, every cell is healed, all the DNA in my body is being transformed by Spirit communicating out loud and being healed." Your crown chakra will be awakened and blessed.

This process I am describing is a constant honoring of the healing that is going on. As you continue saying a blessed mantra or prayer, you are invoking Divine Spirit in the body. Stay in the body with your breath, and you will be breathing in life. The last step is to check the lymph nodes around your throat for any swelling or abnormalities.

Remember that a high-vibration field shields you from negative energies. It can keep your immune system strong, build a strong relationship with the Divine Mother, and give you a daily alignment with Spirit. You will have learned how to be in the God Frequency.

6

5TH DIMENSION CHAKRA-BALANCING SYSTEM

Chakra is a Sanskrit word meaning *wheel, circle, cycle,* or *disk.* Vedic texts also use the word *chakra* in other contexts, such as "wheel of time" or "wheel of dharma."

Dharma is an important term used in several Indian religions. Dharma has no single word equivalent in any Western language. It has many varying meanings, including "cosmic law and order," and encompasses such concepts as duty, rights, vocation, customs, character, law, statute, steadfast decree, justice, virtue, practice, religion, ethics, good work, quality, nature, that which is correct or morally upright, as well as actions necessary for life on an individual and collective basis.

So, when we imagine chakras as wheels of dharma, we can also imagine them as wheels of these and several other qualities.

Because our chakras are embedded within our bodies at various locations, we can see how different points in our bodies are related to our manifestation of the many qualities contained within the concept of dharma. According to the ancient Hindus and Buddhists who researched the spiritual nature of humanity, humans have both a physical body, as well as multiple nonphysical energetic bodies, or subtle bodies, that coexist with the physical body. The chakras are part of our spiritual anatomy.

Chakras are swirling vortices of energy that form junctions between the physical and energetic bodies. Chakras occur at various points along the spine, from the base of the spine to the top of the head. The swirling energy within the chakra is called *prana*. Prana energizes both the physical body and the connected energetic bodies. Prana is transported through the body by a network of channels similar to the arteries that carry blood in the circulatory system. These prana channels are called *nadis*.

The chakras help balance and deliver the proper amount of cosmic energy to your body, mind, and soul, according to your current level of spiritual development. In addition to storing and distributing energy and information, the chakras also serve as the location of our psychological or mental tendencies, habits, desires, and aspects of the subconscious mind. Our inner struggle to grow spiritually takes place between the pull of the soul from above and the pull of the material world from below.

Each chakra manifests different qualities like love, power, or peace. These qualities can manifest positively or negatively, depending on the direction of a person's energy. When we raise our energy inward and upward, we raise our consciousness, which reduces negative qualities, and eventually we attain spiritual liberation.

Here is a list of the chakras and their locations in your body. There are also colors associated with each chakra. The first three chakras are more physical in nature.

Root chakra. The first chakra, at the base of the spine, is red like fire. It represents security and survival. When our consciousness is going downward in this chakra, we become stubborn or too attached to material things. Blockages may appear as fear, paranoia, defensiveness, and procrastination. When we raise our energy up through this chakra, we are more able to concentrate and persevere.

Sacral chakra. The second chakra, just below the navel, is orange like the sun. This chakra represents desire, pleasure, sexuality, procreation, and creativity. Blockage may manifest as emotional problems, obsessive compulsive behavior, and sexual guilt. When we raise our consciousness in this chakra, we become more creative, open-minded, and more receptive to Divine inspiration.

Solar plexus chakra. The third chakra, in the stomach area, is yellow. Feelings of ambition, achievement, personal power, laughter, joy, and anger are associated with this chakra. Blockages in the solar plexus chakra may manifest as anger, frustration, lack of direction, or a feeling of victimization. This chakra's lower form can trigger desires for personal power. In its higher form, the solar plexus chakra increases self-control and willpower so we can achieve what we set our minds to.

Heart chakra. The fourth chakra, in the center of the chest, is green. This chakra is all about love. It is the center of love, peace, harmony, and compassion. In its highest form, this love is all-embracing and unconditional, the love of God. In its negative form, the love becomes restricted to only our own desires.

Throat chakra. The fifth chakra, at the base of the throat, is blue. When our energy is positively oriented, this chakra gives us calmness and inner peace. Blockages can show up as creative blocks, dishonesty, or problems in communicating one's needs to others.

Third eye chakra. The sixth chakra, in the forehead, between the eyebrows, is indigo. This chakra relates to contemplating the spiritual nature of our life. It is the chakra of knowing, perception, inner vision, wisdom, and intuition—even visions of past lives can come through the third eye chakra. Blockages may manifest as lack of foresight, fixed thinking, skepticism, depression, delusions, anxiety, paranoia, vivid dreams, and nightmares.

Crown chakra. The seventh chakra, at the top of the head, is violet. The crown chakra is concerned with understanding, information, acceptance, and bliss. The crown chakra can be said to be your own place of connection to God, the chakra of Divine purpose and personal destiny. It is at the crown chakra where we completely merge with God and achieve final liberation. The crown chakra is usually the last chakra to be awakened. Problems in this chakra can manifest as isolation, loneliness, inability to connect with others, lack of direction, inability to set or maintain goals, and feeling disconnected spiritually. If we look at paintings of Jesus, we can often see a halo around the head. This halo is indicative of his radiant and fully activated crown chakra.

The seven chakras are often referred to as *lotuses* whose petals open in spiritual Awakening. The chakras are like lotus flowers growing from the energetic spine, which is like a flower stem.

We can learn to improve the flow of prana (life) energy through our chakras using various techniques like kriya yoga, taught by the renowned spiritual teacher and yogi Paramahansa Yogananda.

When the chakras are fully opened, or unlocked, enlightenment occurs. This is the goal of all true yoga, including kriya yoga. Yogananda's guru, Swami Sri Yukteswar Giri, compared the chakras to "seven golden candlesticks . . . Seven shining places in the body where the Spirit becomes manifested." Yogananda described the chakras as "seven divinely planned exits or 'trap doors' through which the devotee, by meditation, may escape by seven successive steps into Cosmic Consciousness."

5TH DIMENSIONAL CHAKRA-BALANCING EXERCISES FOR SELF-HEALING

For empowering, healing, and forgiving.

Getting into Position

First, we will assume a meditative pose.

If you are able to sit with your legs crossed, also called lotus style, this is recommended. If you are not able to sit cross-legged, there are other meditative poses you can use, such as lying down—called Savasana—or even sitting in a chair with your feet flat on the floor. No matter which pose you use, try to keep your spine straight and aligned with your neck and head.

If sitting, try to sit on a surface that will be comfortable for several minutes. You can even sit on a pillow, a cushion, a sofa, a bed, or a meditation chair. You can place pillows behind your back to help support your spine if needed. Try to sit as upright as possible, with a straight spine. You should feel comfortable and relaxed. You should not feel pain. Pain will distract your meditation and should be avoided. If you feel pain, adjust yourself so that you are comfortable. If needed, switch to a more comfortable meditation pose. Sitting lotus-style becomes easier with practice and stretching exercises.

If sitting, place your hands on your knees or in your lap, with palms turned upward in a relaxed manner.

If you are lying down, lie flat on your back on a comfortable surface. Keep your arms at your sides. Turn your palms so they face upward in a relaxed manner. You can place a pillow underneath your knees and/or head if it makes you more comfortable. Your body should feel completely at rest. This lying-down pose is called Savasana.

Aligning Your Hands

Now, whether sitting or lying down, place your thumbs against your index or middle fingers. This is called a *mudra*. A mudra is a hand gesture used during meditation to channel the body's energy flow. There are over one hundred mudras. Different mudras modulate your energy flow in different ways and have different effects.

Prana mudra is a powerful mudra that helps channel and focus prana energy, which is the energetic force that flows through your chakras. Prana mudra is perfect for working with the prana energy of the chakras.

Here's how to do prana mudra: First, make a peace sign with your fingers. Then bring your index and middle fingers together. You are now performing prana mudra.

The Chakra-Balancing Exercise

To start, close your eyes.

Take three deep breaths.

As you inhale and exhale slowly and steadily, tap your

crown chakra three times. Your crown chakra is located on the top of your head. This chakra is the universal chakra of God. The crown chakra is your own place of connection to God, the chakra of Divine purpose and personal destiny. The crown chakra is often represented with the color violet or white.

Slowly tap the top of your head three times as you draw the energy of Spirit into your crown chakra. Feel the wonder of the current of the energy flow as the spirits heal you.

Through your breath, you are drawing in the energy of Spirit into your crown chakra, emanating the color violet or white.

Continuing to move down the body, we will now activate your third eye chakra, which helps awaken your intuition. The third eye is represented by the color indigo.

Take three deep breaths.

As you inhale and exhale slowly and steadily, tap your third eye chakra three times, right between your eyebrows. This is where your third eye chakra is located. The third eye itself is located just above this point.

Focus on the color indigo to help awaken your third eye.

Next, we will open the throat chakra. The throat chakra helps with clear communication. It is represented by the color blue.

Take three deep breaths to open the throat chakra while envisioning the color blue.

Then say, "I am strong, I am love, I am healed."

Now swallow.

Continuing to move down the body, we will now activate your heart chakra, which helps awaken your intuition.

Located in the center of your chest, the heart chakra represents your ability to love unconditionally. The heart chakra is represented by the color green.

Breathing deeply and slowly, bring your hand over your heart three times with love and compassion.

As you continue to sit or lie flat, rub both of your hands together, heating up your palms.

As you inhale and exhale slowly and steadily, tap your hands to your solar plexus chakra three times, which is located two inches above your navel. The solar plexus chakra helps improve the expression of will and personal power. This chakra is represented by the color yellow.

Picture a golden rope connecting to your solar plexus as you become one with the Omnipresent.

The sacral chakra is located three inches below the navel, at the center of your lower belly. The sacral chakra is associated with emotions, feelings, sexuality, and creativity. The sacral chakra is represented by the color orange.

As you inhale and exhale slowly and steadily, tap your hands to your sacral chakra three times. Breathe in as the Spirit Guides heal your sacral chakra. Focus on feeling harmony as love permeates your body.

To heal your sacral chakra, say out loud, "The spirits have healed my sacral chakra because I live in forgiveness. I forgive everyone in my sacral chakra."

As you inhale and exhale slowly and steadily, tap your hands to your root chakra three times. The root chakra is located at the base of your spine, encompassing the pelvic floor. The root chakra is responsible for your sense of safety and security. The root chakra is represented by the color red. Envision a beautiful red rose petal.

Now shout out loud, "Love! Love! Love! Love! Love!" as you invoke the energy of healing, aligning your root chakra.

Red jasper and tourmaline can be helpful crystals for healing of the root chakra.

Selenite and rose quartz are also very helpful crystals for healing and working with the chakras.

Self-Protection Chakra Closing Seal

After we open our chakras to receive energy, it is important that we seal our chakras to preserve the energy we have received. This will give you more energy in your daily life. If we don't seal our chakras, we may feel that we have lost energy.

Begin by taking three deep breaths. With a softly closed hand, touch all your chakras in the same order as you began, beginning with the crown chakra and moving down. This seals in the energy.

Finally, place a 12th Dimensional Shield all around your entire body. This helps keep your chakras in balance for longer periods of time.

After you have completed the exercise, you can lie down with a gemstone placed on each chakra and meditate.

Using music and gemstones is always helpful with the exercise.

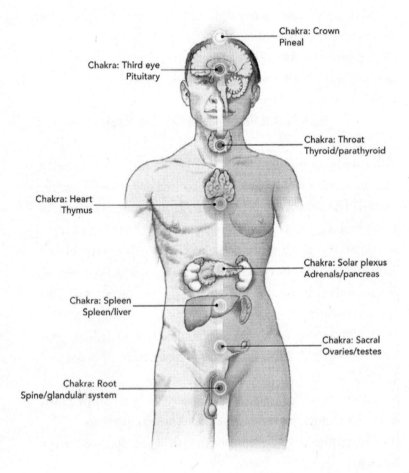

5TH DIMENSION MIND AND BODY:

PRACTICES FOR HEALING

5th Dimension healing requires us to strengthen our souls, our minds, and our bodies.

In addition to the spiritual practices, there are other ways we can raise our bodies' vibration so that we are experiencing the 5th Dimension as much as possible. Remember, it is in the 5th Dimension that we can experience rapid healing.

The following chapters contain information, practices, and exercises that will lift your body's vibration, which can help with healing. It's important to nourish not just our Spirit but also our minds and bodies, so that we are surrounding ourselves with the highest practices that we may have the highest experiences.

Read through the chapters, and then go back and highlight those ideas and practices that you feel will raise your vibration.

In this chapter, you'll find:

The 5th Dimension Lifestyle Healing Agreements

Supplements and Therapy Suggestions

Superfoods List

Medical Intuitive Nutritional Meal Plans

Omnivorous Food Plan Outline

Vegetarian Food Plan Outline

Vegan Food Plan Outline

Immune-Boosting Shakes

The 5D List of Health Dos and Don'ts

7

WATER CAN
SAVE YOUR LIFE

Water is a 5th Dimension substance. Every day, we drink water, and it's essential to our health that we consume only the most natural and highest-quality water available to us. Most medical conditions are triggered, in some way, by drinking contaminated water. I feel it's most important to make sure that we're highly informed, and this is information that I share with all of my healing clients.

Water covers 70 percent of Earth's surface, and it's even found in deep outer space. The constituent atoms of water, or H_2O, are hydrogen and oxygen, the first- and third-most common elements throughout the Universe. Water is also known as "the universal solvent" because more chemicals dissolve in water than in any other substance.

Water is vital for life. The human body is composed of 60 to 70 percent water, and without it, humans die within a few days. In cases of extreme heat, death for want of water can come within hours. All cells—whether human, animal, or plant—require water to perform their functions. Within the body, water performs multiple general yet critical roles: chemical reaction medium, temperature regulator, transportation vehicle, lubricant, and shock absorber. Because water is the universal solvent, it can also help flush toxins from the body via urine and stool, thanks to the work of the liver and kidneys, which both filter toxins from the blood.

It makes sense that life is so dependent on this amazing molecule! But the *quality* of the water we take into our bodies is also of critical importance. Because water is such a good solvent, it can easily absorb chemicals that are harmful to humans, animals, and plants. This means if the water we drink is contaminated, the contamination can be carried into and absorbed by our bodies! Not good! Unfortunately, countless people around the world suffer many kinds of sickness—and even death—that can be linked to environmental toxins. This is why toxin-free water, food, shelter, air, and land are central to a long life of health and vitality.

EARTH'S POLLUTION PROBLEM

Chief Seattle said, "Man did not weave this web of life. He is merely a strand in it. Whatever he does to the web, he does to himself."

Sadly, humanity has done a great deal to disrupt the web of life on Earth—and in doing so, we are hurting not only our fellow earthlings but ourselves as well. One manifestation of this damage comes in the form of pollution. There are few regions of the earth unspoiled and unharmed by some form of pollution. The forms of pollution are vast, the costs to lives and health are high, and the potential outcomes look increasingly dire.

This pollution problem has also significantly and negatively affected the quality of much of the earth's water, including ground and well water, municipal water supplies, and even the world's oceans. All countries and all oceans are affected in some way. In the United States alone, almost half of all rivers and streams, and more than one-third of all lakes, are so polluted that they are unsafe for swimming, fishing, or drinking.

Pollutants can include sewage, petrochemicals like plastics, industrial and agricultural wastes, pesticides, Bisphenol-A (BPA, a resin that leaches out of plastic bottles and causes cancer), and even prescription medications like birth control hormones and antidepressants. Heavy metals are also a real problem. Mercury, arsenic, lead, copper, and cadmium and other toxic heavy metals can all cause significant health issues, including cancer, disorders of the reproductive and nervous systems, and damage to the vital organs, including the brain. Heavy metal contamination can come from sources like agricultural and industrial operations, power plants (especially coal-fired), sewage, mining, and even water pipes in houses.

Radiation in water is also a concern. According to a study by the Environmental Working Group, more than 170 million Americans—from all fifty states—drink radioactive water. Radioactivity can lead to cancer and fetal developmental problems. Water that may pass the Environmental Protection Agency's old standards set in 1976 can fail newer, more stringent standards set by California state scientists in 2006.

PROTECT OURSELVES FROM PLASTICS

Modern civilization has a voracious appetite for plastic. Most humans use plastic, and we're producing more than ever, making it a major pollution problem.

Plastics are made of thousands of chemicals, many of which can mimic human hormones and disrupt the human endocrine system. The consequences of overexposure to some of these chemicals can include cancers, birth defects, damaged immunity, developmental and reproductive effects, metabolism problems, and insulin resistance.

It's perhaps impossible for you to avoid plastics entirely, but reducing your exposure and risk profile is possible—and necessary—to help protect your health. Consuming foods or liquids that have been stored in plastic containers should be avoided as much as possible, especially if the container has been bent, dented, creased, crushed, crumpled, or left in the sun. Different plastics have different properties and present different risks. The safest plastic is no plastic.

Containers made from high-temperature glass are ideal. High-temperature glass is safer than regular glass. Food-grade stainless steel would be the second option. Copper containers may be used occasionally but not every day. Copper is necessary for good health, but too much is toxic.

Try to find a good source of clean tested mountain spring

water, as I recommend in the following chapters and in the resource guide.

Bathing and showering present unique challenges. Showerheads can aerosolize chlorine—another toxin to be avoided—as well as bacteria and molds, such as aspergillus, which could cause significant illness to someone with a compromised immune system. A high-quality shower filter head is recommended for showering. For bathing, a chlorine filtering bath ball is recommended.

By drinking high-quality water, you are oxygenating your body and accelerating the healing process. Pure water is a blessing for all life on this planet. It is impossible for life to function without it.

Water is a gift from God.

8

5TH DIMENSION BODY—HEALTHY NUTRITIONAL PRACTICES

This chapter contains many ideas, lists, exercises, food plans, and even recipes that can help you lift your body's vibrational pattern to the 5th Dimension. This is meant to be a good overview for you, to give you an idea of how you can best support your body, which in turn helps you to support your mind and soul. We can't only be in alignment spiritually, we need to align our body and mind with the 5th Dimension.

Up to 85 percent of the people I scan are immune suppressed to one extent or another. To recover from any serious immune-suppressed condition, including viruses or cancer, requires a serious commitment from you. While God can heal, you must be open to accepting the healing. You must welcome your healing by providing it a healthy home within your heart, mind, body, and Spirit. Regaining your health requires a willingness to modify habits and become open to new, healthier ways of living.

In addition to having a sincere relationship with God, there are other practices you can consistently engage in to root yourself in a vibratory state of high consciousness. In the following protocols, which are the same ones I give to my Healing Trilogy clients, you will find ways to boost your immune system and oxygenate the body to help support your healing process.

Many people come to me in a weakened state after having been encouraged to experiment with detoxification. These detox techniques include coffee enemas, apple cider vinegar, and turmeric. In my experience, detoxification, as currently practiced, weakens the immune system.

Needless to say, I am a firm believer in boosting the immune system, rather than detoxing, especially if my clients are already immune suppressed. Eating only fruits and vegetables can result in dehydration and can cause rapid loss of weight, while having high levels of sugar and low levels of oxygen in the body suppresses the immune system.

The health advice I give to clients comes from a combination of guidance I receive from a high level of Spirit, from scanning some of the latest scientific literature, and from observing patterns in the hundreds of clients I have worked with over the years. My approach is similar to that of a private investigator, doing diagnostics for early detection, and then giving clients a preventative list of ways to boost their immune system and protect it from toxins.

During the time I spend with each client, I ask them questions about such things as what kind of water they are drinking and bathing in, are they vitamin D suppressed (the vitamin that the sun provides), what they eat, what kind of herbs and supplements and medications they are on, and the nature of their relationship to Spirit. Then I do their body scan, which brings up even more information. I blink in codes to reveal the needs of clients, and I answer their questions with coded blinking.

From the patterns of evidence that I have collected, I created these categories of recommendations that I give those in need of healing to accompany their entry into 5th Dimensional states of consciousness.

Read through the following pages first, and then go back and start creating your own 5D health plan.

THE 5TH DIMENSION LIFESTYLE
HEALING AGREEMENTS

Let's start with the Lifestyle Healing Agreements, within which you can structure your prevention and healing experience. Each of the agreements in this list is what I often ask my clients to agree to in lifting their vibration into the 5th Dimension.

Go through this list, and check the ones that resonate with you. Remember that before you start or stop any program, consult with your health care practitioner.

My Lifestyle Healing Agreements Checklist

- Agree to refrain from smoking.
- Agree to refrain from abusing illicit or prescription drugs.
- Agree to avoid detoxification methods that involve coffee enemas. Healing comes through boosting of the immune system, and detoxification can suppress the immune system because essential minerals get removed from the body through dehydration.
- Agree to avoid use of heating pads.
- Agree to live in a clean home environment while healing.
- Agree to get plenty of rest, at least eight hours of sleep per night.
- Agree to avoid apple cider vinegar, which causes esophageal and intestinal stress.
- Agree to avoid turmeric and curcumin extracts, because they inflame the body.
- Agree to avoid steam rooms, saunas, spas, Jacuzzis, and so on. This includes avoiding the steam from a shower as much as possible. The water from the steam can suppress your immune system. You might also be breathing in chlorine, which is not healthy.
- Agree to avoid bathing in chlorinated water. All showers should have a chlorine filter. All bathtubs should have a chlorine filter. (See the appendix for specific brands I recommend.)
- Agree to avoid exposure to mold.

- Agree to protect yourself against toxic air with a HEPA air filter, such as Honeywell.
- Agree to AVOID DRINKING FROM ANY PLASTIC BOTTLES. Instead, drink from glass or food-grade steel. Almost all plastics leach chemicals, like BPA, that disrupt your endocrine system. See this link for a good explanation of the safety of various plastics: https://www.glutathionediseasecure .com/safe-plastics.html.
- Agree to avoid stress, because stress lowers the immune system.
- Agree to chant, pray, or meditate at least five minutes a day to raise consciousness into a higher Dimension.
- Agree to seek laughter and happiness and joy, as these boost the immune system and open the heart as well.
- Agree to get twenty minutes of full-body sunshine a day.
- Agree to refrain from drinking alcohol because it is high in sugar.
- Agree to avoid all soy.
- Agree to avoid bananas and oranges and other high-sugar tropical fruits. Blueberries, blackberries, and raspberries may be enjoyed instead.
- Agree to consume more raw organic honey, which is healthy and delicious. (Organic honey is a natural antibiotic and a high-quality sweetener that

contains trace minerals, as opposed to table sugar, which has no nutritional value.)

- Agree to avoid consuming sugary foods, a.k.a. junk food, including desserts, candy, juices, sodas, and so on, because they feed cancer.

- Agree to avoid foods that have a high-glycemic index, such as white breads, pastries, potatoes, white sugar, white rice, bran flakes, corn flakes, and tropical fruits.

- Agree to eat foods that have a LOW SCORE on the glycemic index, such as sweet potatoes, oat bran, quinoa, and vegetables.

- Agree to avoid eating fish or marine creatures, including shark, swordfish, shellfish, and crustaceans like shrimp, lobsters, clams, and oysters, because many studies have found that there are toxic pollutants in fish across the world's oceans.

- Agree to eat fresh, healthy, whole, living, unprocessed, unpackaged, freshly prepared plant-based foods as much as possible.

- If eating meat, agree to eat grass-fed organic meat raised humanely.

- Agree to drink lots of pure spring water from a container made of glass or food-grade stainless steel. Copper may be used occasionally but not daily. (See the appendix for my specific recommendations.)

SUPPLEMENTS AND THERAPY SUGGESTIONS

Many people ask me what supplements they should take and what other treatments I recommend to increase their bodies' vibrations. The following is a general list of supplements and therapies that I often recommend. *The quantities and concentrations are general, and you should work with your health care practitioner to determine the proper amounts and combinations for you, or take as directed on the item's package.*

See appendix 1, "5th Dimension Resources," for more information on these.

- Dr. Shealy's Biogenics Magnesium Lotion and Magnesium Lotion Spray
- U-Tract Complete by Progressive Laboratories (for urinary tract)
- G5 Siliplant (ingestible liquid)
- Silicium G5 gel (topical)
- Inner-ēco coconut probiotic (plain)—(for digestive health)—I often suggest to clients to take one ounce every day to boost your immune system.
- 1 oz. wheatgrass shots—twice a week or more. Available from any good natural foods store or juice store, or you can grow it at home.
- Ozonated water—can be made at home with an ozone machine and a bubbler. Ozonate water for ten to twenty minutes. Consume within ten minutes, as ozone will dissipate quickly.

- Hyperbaric oxygen therapy—requires a doctor's prescription
- Vitamin K2, zinc, and boron
- Fish-free, algae-based omega acid EPA and DHA supplement
- Multivitamin
- B-6 and B-12 100 mg veggie caps
- D3 5,000 IU
- Selenium
- Lysine
- GABA for anxiety
- Blessed Ormus Cream

PREVENTION AND TREATMENT USING SUPERFOODS

There are a few foods I have singled out for special recognition. These superfoods offer some very important nutrients that can power-pack your meals and snacks and further enhance a healthy eating pattern.

MY SUPERFOODS LIST

- Berries. Blueberries, blackberries, raspberries. High in fiber, berries are naturally sweet, and their rich colors mean they are high in antioxidants and disease-fighting nutrients.
- Eggs. The best protein source on the planet, eggs beat out milk, whey, and soy in the pro-

tein they provide. Please eat the yolk. The yolk contains choline, which helps protect heart and brain functions and prevents cholesterol and fats from accumulating in the liver. Also drinking half a glass a day of beet root juice helps detox the liver and acts as an anti-inflammatory.

- Leafy greens. Dark, leafy greens are a good source of vitamin A, vitamin C, and calcium, as well as several phytochemicals (chemicals made by plants that have a positive effect on your health). They also add fiber into the diet. How to include them: Try varieties such as spinach, swiss chard, kale, collard greens, or mustard greens. Throw them into salads or sauté them in a little olive oil. You can also add greens to soups and stews.

- Olive oil. Olive oil is a good source of vitamin E, polyphenols, and monounsaturated fatty acids, all of which help reduce the risk of heart disease. How to include it: Use in place of butter or margarine in pasta or rice dishes. Drizzle over vegetables, use as a dressing, or when sautéing.

- Whole grains. A good source of both soluble and insoluble fiber, whole grains also contain several B vitamins, minerals, and phytonutrients. They have been shown to lower cholesterol and protect against heart disease and diabetes. How to include them: Try having a bowl of oatmeal for breakfast. Substitute bulgur, quinoa, wheat berries or brown rice, and sweet potatoes. When buying bread at the supermarket, check to see that the first ingredient is "100 percent whole wheat flour."

- Yogurt. A good source of calcium and protein, yogurt also contains live cultures called *probiotics.* These good bacteria can protect the body from other, more harmful bacteria. Remember to buy plain yogurt and add your own fruit. Look for yogurts that have live active cultures, such as *Lactobacillus, L. acidophilus, L. bulgaricus,* and *S. thermophilus.* Remember to stay away from low-fat labels. You can use yogurt in place of mayonnaise or sour cream in dips or sauces. Too much yogurt is not advised in place of a probiotic.

- Cruciferous vegetables. These include broccoli, avocado, brussels sprouts, cabbage, cauliflower, collard greens, asparagus, kale, kohlrabi, mustard greens, radishes, and turnips. They are an excellent source of fiber, vitamins, and phytochemicals including indoles, thiocyanates, and nitriles, which may prevent some types of cancer. How to include them: Steam or stir-fry, adding healthy olive oil, coconut oil, and herbs and seasonings for flavor. Try adding a frozen cruciferous vegetable medley to soups, casseroles, and pasta dishes.

- Legumes. This broad category includes kidney, black, red, and garbanzo beans, as well as soybeans and peas. Legumes are an excellent source of fiber, folate, and plant-based protein. Studies show they can help reduce the risk of heart disease.

- Flaxseed is a great source of fiber that can be used as an anti-inflammatory, and Gandhi himself proclaimed its healing effects. I used it in my recovery; it has tremendous fatty acids and minerals like magnesium, potassium, and zinc.
- Tart cherry juice can reduce inflammation from osteoarthritis (OA) and gout. It reduces muscle soreness and strengthens the immune system.
- Pomegranates contain three times more antioxidants than red wine and green tea do. Green tea is also highly beneficial as an antioxidant; it is an amazing antidote to artery-clogging plaque, which promotes heart disease and stroke. Drinking one glass a day long-term helps slow the aging process and protect against cancer.
- Mushrooms like maitake help prevent and treat cancer, viral disease, high cholesterol, and high blood pressure. Also, studies show consuming mushrooms can lower cholesterol 45 percent. I have seen this to be true.

MEDICAL INTUITIVE NUTRITIONAL MEAL PLANS

Every day, people ask me what they should eat and in which food combinations.

Whether they describe themselves as vegan, vegetarian, or plant-based, I tell them I don't think it's healthy to just have a shake all the time and call it a meal. Even many of my vegans are going back to eating a little bit of protein, such as eggs. I am not an advocate of killing animals. Some of my clients are in poor health and they will benefit from eating an egg. To be clear, it's okay to eat an egg. Egg whites are a healthy source of protein, especially if you have fatty liver.

Ideally, all the food and beverages you consume should be organic. You don't want to be putting pesticide and herbicide residues into your body. Also, during meal prep, this is important: for any foods you need to rinse off, you must use filtered water, not tap water.

Please note the following lists contain items that are suitable for those who adhere to various dietary lifestyles. Vegetarians and vegans are offered many options in the lists below and are asked to kindly disregard any suggested food they are not comfortable eating.

Beverages

- Mountain Valley spring water, or any quality spring water. (Water should not be stored in plastic. Drinking water should not come from underground wells or municipal sources.)
- Those on a renal diet or receiving dialysis should consult with their medical provider as to what kind of water they should be drinking.
- Water infused with organic cucumber slices.
- Water infused with sliced fruit.
- Organic coffee.
- Organic tea, black and herbal.

Sweeteners

- Sweeteners should be used sparingly. Some sweeteners are healthier than others.
- Healthier sweeteners: organic natural sweeteners like raw organic honey and organic stevia.
- Less healthy sweeteners: Artificial sweeteners and corn-based sweeteners—I don't recommend these.

Let's Talk About Salad!

- Think of a salad as an opportunity for the healthiest foods in your house to come together and have a party that culminates in your mouth.
- You can experiment with different types of greens to achieve different flavors. Try to move beyond iceberg lettuce, which doesn't have much nutritional value. You can even use a variety of different greens, such as arugula, swiss chard, mustard greens, kale, spinach, dandelion greens, and so on.
- *Salad toppings*: tomatoes, dill, rosemary, goji berries, pomegranate seeds, hemp seeds, chia seeds, blueberries, blackberries, boysenberries, grapes, peaches, pears, nectarines, mangoes, apples.
- You can also add fresh organic herbs like parsley, sage, rosemary, thyme (just like the song), plus dill, mint, lemon balm, basil, oregano, chives, coriander, cilantro, and the like.
- Boost your nutrition with microgreens; microgreens are a great way to add nutrients to any meal or smoothie.

- Nutritious microgreens include wheatgrass, watercress, alfalfa sprouts, sunflower sprouts, pea sprouts, clover sprouts, and lentil sprouts.

OMNIVOROUS FOOD PLAN OUTLINE

Breakfast—Organic

- Fresh, free-range eggs (up to two), whole-grain oatmeal, yogurt, hormone-free turkey or chicken, avocado, manna bread
- Seasonal fruit not high in sugar, including blueberries, blackberries, raspberries, peaches, pears, Granny Smith apples, mango, and gluten-free pancakes. (Eat all in moderation.)

Lunch—Organic

- Hormone-free turkey or chicken, avocado, manna bread
- Quinoa with sweet potatoes and chicken and spinach
- Arugula, avocado, pecans
- Brussels sprouts
- Shiitake mushrooms
- Portobello mushrooms
- Soups: asparagus, broccoli, tomato, sweet potato, chicken bone broth, beef bone broth, turkey bone broth, homemade chicken soup

Snacks—Organic

- Try to have a Granny Smith apple daily.
- Afternoon smoothie (see recipes below)

Dinner—Organic

- Any protein, such as turkey breast or chicken or beef. (My Guides suggest beef no more than once a week if a meat eater.)
- Avocados. (Eat one a day as a great source of protein.)
- Vegetables (spinach no more than twice a week)
- Soups (fresh, not canned soups)
  - Turkey or chicken vegetable noodle with wild rice
  - French onion
  - Broccoli
- Lentils
- Quinoa, turkey, organic ground beef
- Gluten-free pasta
- Wild rice
- Vegetable stir-fry
- Wilted kale salad
- Squash
- Artichokes
- Sweet potato
- Zucchini
- Meat and vegetable pot pie

RECIPES

Here are some recipes that I recommend. Please feel free to augment these recipes to fit your tastes.

Organic Meat Loaf Dinner

INGREDIENTS:
- 1 pound ground turkey
- 1 pound grass-fed ground beef
- 2 large eggs
- $\frac{1}{2}$ cup cooked quinoa
- 2 teaspoons unrefined sea salt
- $\frac{1}{8}$ teaspoon black pepper
- 1 small onion, finely diced
- 2 cloves garlic, minced
- $\frac{1}{2}$ cup raw milk or coconut milk

FOR THE SAUCE:
- 3 oz. organic tomato paste
- $1\frac{1}{2}$ tablespoons raw honey
- 1 tablespoon yellow mustard
- 2 tablespoons water
- $\frac{1}{8}$ teaspoon unrefined sea salt

DIRECTIONS:
1. Preheat oven to 350 degrees.
2. To make sauce, add all of the sauce ingredients to a bowl and whisk until well combined.
3. Combine all meat loaf ingredients and mix until well blended. Shape into a loaf.
4. Place meat loaf into a loaf pan and pour the sauce on top (we like a lot of sauce on our meat loaf, so I double the sauce recipe).
5. Bake for 1 hour and 15 minutes.

Kimberly's Seasoned Chicken Recipe

INGREDIENTS:

6–8 skinless, boneless organic chicken thighs
1 to 2 bunches asparagus or broccoli
1 tablespoon lemon juice
5 cloves garlic, chopped
Italian herbs like oregano, thyme, and rosemary
Kosher salt
Freshly ground black pepper
5 sprigs mint
1 teaspoon honey
Sliced lemons

DIRECTIONS:

1. Preheat oven to 400 degrees. Line a baking sheet with parchment paper. Arrange chicken and broccoli or asparagus on the baking sheet.
2. In a small bowl, combine the lemon juice and chopped garlic and herbs. Season with salt and pepper.
3. Coat the chicken and asparagus or broccoli in the baking sheet with the lemon juice and herbs, then place in the oven.
4. Bake for 30 minutes.
5. Serve immediately.

Kale Salad

1. Suitable for all, including vegetarians and vegans.

INGREDIENTS:

Extra-virgin olive oil
2 garlic cloves, minced
1 bunch kale, cut into bite-size pieces
Dried cranberries
Organic walnuts

FOR THE VINAIGRETTE:
  1 tablespoon extra-virgin olive oil
  ½ teaspoon dijon mustard
  Pepper and sea salt

DIRECTIONS:
  1. Heat the olive oil and add garlic. Sauté until the garlic is fragrant. Add the kale and sauté until wilted. Remove from the heat.
  2. Whisk the vinaigrette ingredients together.
  3. Add the cranberries and the walnuts to the wilted kale. Drizzle with the vinaigrette and serve warm.

VEGETARIAN FOOD PLAN OUTLINE

Ideally, all of the food you consume should be organic.

A few words about meat alternatives. Many meat alternatives contain soy. I do not recommend consuming soy because most soy is genetically modified. Tofu, tempeh, and textured vegetable protein all contain soy. Seitan is made from wheat gluten. Seitan may work for some, but those who are sensitive to gluten, or those who have irritable bowel syndrome or celiac disease, will want to avoid seitan.

Numerous other meat alternatives exist, including Beyond Meat and Impossible Foods, though I generally don't recommend Impossible Foods because it contains genetically modified ingredients. These items currently should not be thought of as health foods. But they are healthier than the animal meat they are replacing, and they are generally better for the environment. Some brands are healthier than others. Dr. Praeger's veggie burgers are on the healthier side.

Breakfast—Organic Vegetarian

- Fresh, organic, free-range eggs (up to two eggs), whole-grain oatmeal, quinoa (or teff) breakfast bowl, yogurt, blueberries, blackberries, strawberries, goji berries, apples, pears, peaches, avocado, manna bread (may be unsuitable for those with gluten intolerance, celiac disease, or leaky gut), flaxseeds, hemp seeds
- Vegetarian eggs benedict on manna bread
- Vegan scramble
- Your favorite delicious protein shake
- Seasonal fruit, but not those high in sugar

Quinoa Alternative

Quinoa is great, but another gluten-free grain worthy of your consideration is teff, an ancient grain from Africa. For thousands of years, teff has been eaten in Ethiopia and Eritrea. Several world-record-holding runners from Africa consume teff as a staple part of their training diet. Remarkably, teff is the only grain to supply vitamin C. In fact, one serving can supply the recommended minimum daily intake of vitamin C. Teff also supplies protein and other nutrients, including calcium, magnesium, zinc, and B vitamins. Thanks to its resistant starch content, teff is low on the glycemic index, helping with blood sugar stabilization and weight maintenance. The intestinal microbiome benefits when you consume this grain, which is the world's tiniest. It can be eaten as a porridge for breakfast, or made into a big spongy fermented flatbread called injera, which tastes similar to sourdough bread. Traditionally, injera is used to scoop up and eat other foods. You can also use injera to make healthy wraps.

CLOSE UP: 5D HEALTHY BOWLS

Basically, these are bowls of healthy ingredients that taste great together. Depending on the ingredients you used, 5D Healthy Bowls can be eaten any time of day, for breakfast, lunch, or dinner.

Start with a base of cooked grain, such as oatmeal, quinoa, or teff.

Add your favorite healthy, delicious ingredients that pair well together. Below are some ingredients you can consider in creating your own bowls.

Enjoy!

Popular 5D Healthy Bowl Combinations

Sweet 5D Healthy Bowls:

- Apples, cinnamon, seeds or nuts (optional)
- Chai spices
- Optional organic milk, almond milk, oat milk
- Soy milk is not recommended

Savory 5D Healthy Bowls:

- Pesto, avocado, and egg
- Spinach, mushroom, and egg
- Sweet potatoes, egg, bell peppers, onion (optional)
- Egg, cilantro, tomato, avocado, and lemon or lime juice
  (Herbs, salt, and pepper to taste)

Lunch—Organic Vegetarian

- Avocado, manna bread or injera, tomatoes
- Quinoa, sweet potatoes, spinach, arugula, pecans
- Brussels sprouts
- Shiitake mushrooms
- Portobello mushrooms
- Soups: asparagus, broccoli

Snack—Organic

- Afternoon smoothie

Dinner—Organic Vegetarian

- Organic soups: lentil, broccoli, rosemary potato-leek, tomato
- Vegetarian chili
- Quinoa
- Gluten-free pasta

- Lentils
- Wild rice
- Vegetable stir-fry
- Wilted kale salad
- Squash
- Artichokes
- Sweet potato
- Zucchini
- Vegetable pot pie
- Vegetarian shepherd's pie
- Vegetarian lasagna
- A variety of healthy meat alternatives now exist for vegetarians, which taste good and seem very similar to meat.

Vegetarian Meat Loaf Dinner

INGREDIENTS:

2 cups water
1 teaspoon salt
1 cup lentils
1 small onion, diced
1 cup quick-cooking oats
¾ cup Monterey jack or American cheese
1 egg, beaten
4 oz. spaghetti sauce or 4½ oz. tomato sauce
1 teaspoon garlic powder
1 teaspoon dried basil
1 tablespoon dried parsley
1 teaspoon seasoning salt
1 teaspoon black pepper

DIRECTIONS:

1. Preheat the oven to 350 degrees F.
2. Place the water in a saucepan, add the salt, and bring to a boil. Add the lentils and simmer, covered, 25–30 minutes, until the lentils are soft and most of the water has evaporated. Remove from the heat.
3. Drain and partially mash the lentils. Scrape into a mixing bowl and allow to cool slightly. Stir in the onion, oats, and cheese and mix until blended. Add the egg, spaghetti sauce, garlic powder, basil, parsley, seasoning salt, and pepper. Mix well. Spoon into a loaf pan that has been generously sprayed with Pam (nonstick cooking spray). Smooth the top with the back of the spoon.
4. Bake at 350 degrees for 30–45 minutes, until the top is dry, firm, and golden brown.
5. Remove from the oven and let cool in the pan on a cooling rack for about 10 minutes, then serve.

VEGAN FOOD PLAN OUTLINE

Breakfast—Organic Vegan

- Whole-grain oatmeal, quinoa breakfast bowl, blueberries, blackberries, apples, peaches, pears, avocado, manna bread, flaxseeds, hemp seeds
- Your favorite delicious protein shake
- Seasonal fruit not high in sugar

Lunch—Organic Vegan

- Avocado, manna bread
- Quinoa with sweet potatoes and spinach, arugula, avocado, pecans

- Brussels sprouts
- Shiitake mushrooms
- Portobello mushrooms
- Soups: asparagus, broccoli
- Kale salad
- Quinoa
- Gluten-free pasta
- Lentils
- Wild rice
- Vegetable stir-fry
- Squash
- Artichokes
- Sweet potato
- Zucchini

Snack—Organic

- Afternoon smoothie (see recipes below)

Dinner—Organic Vegan

- Organic extra-virgin olive oil
- Pure coconut oil
- Baked sweet potatoes
- Organic soups: broccoli, mixed vegetable, vegan black bean chili
- Quinoa
- Gluten-free pasta
- Lentils

- Wild rice
- Vegetable stir-fry
- Wilted kale salad
- Squash
- Artichokes
- Zucchini
- Vegetable pot pie
- Vegan shepherd's pie
- Vegan lasagna

Vegan Egg Scramble

These vegan scrambled eggs are made with chickpea flour instead of tofu for a filling and high-protein breakfast scramble.

INGREDIENTS:
  1 teaspoon olive oil
  ½ onion, chopped
  1 medium tomato, chopped
  1½ cups (4 oz./113 g) sliced mushrooms

FOR THE VEGAN SCRAMBLE MIX:
  ½ cup (46 g) chickpea flour
  ½ cup (120 ml) oat milk (or flax milk or almond milk)
  2 tablespoons nutritional yeast
  1 teaspoon dijon mustard
  ½ teaspoon garlic powder
  ¼ teaspoon black salt (Kala Namak)
  ¼ teaspoon onion powder
  Sundried tomatoes
  Add any veggie you'd like

DIRECTIONS:

1. Combine all Vegan Scramble Mix ingredients in a bowl, whisk until well mixed, and set aside.
2. In a skillet, add the olive oil, tomato, onion, mushrooms along with any additional veggies you would like. Cook over medium heat until onions are soft, about five minutes.
3. Add the contents of the bowl into the skillet, and cook, stirring occasionally until consistency is like scrambled eggs.

Wild Rice Soup

1. For winter or summer, wild rice soup is so comforting for the soul.
2. This wild rice soup is creamy, it's cozy, it's savory: it's made 100 percent of plants. Yes, this is vegan wild rice soup.
3. *This is really the best soup ever.*
4. While it takes about 1 hour to make, this is super healthy and 100 percent worth the effort. And since most of that time is hands off, it's easy.
5. Use cashews. Blended cashews can stand in for dairy! In this wild rice soup, you'll let them soak while the soup simmers. Then you'll take 2 cups of the soup out (veggies and all) and blend it with the soaked cashews. It cleans the nuts and makes for the creamiest base EVER. You'll swear there's dairy in it.
6. Add white beans and mushrooms. This wild rice soup features white beans as a plant-based protein. It's a unique addition and seriously good. Mushrooms also bring in big flavor and texture.
7. Simmer until the rice pops. Wild rice notoriously takes quite a while to cook: upward of 50 minutes. You'll cook this soup until most of the rice grains burst and are tender. It might feel like a long time, but it's important that the rice be perfectly tender.

INGREDIENTS:

(Quinoa can be substituted for wild rice.)

½ cup organic cashews

1 medium yellow onion

2 celery stalks

3 medium carrots

8 oz. baby bella mushrooms

6 cloves garlic

2 tablespoons olive oil

1 tablespoon dried thyme

1 tablespoon dried oregano

8 cups vegetable broth

1 cup wild rice (not a wild rice blend)

2 teaspoons kosher salt, divided

2 15-ounce cans white beans, drained and rinsed

½ teaspoon black pepper

2 teaspoons dried sage

1 tablespoon liquid amino acids

DIRECTIONS:

1. Place the raw cashews in a bowl and cover them with water. Leave them to soak while you make the soup.

2. Dice the onion. Thinly slice the celery. Cut the carrots into rounds. Slice the mushrooms. Mince the garlic.

3. Place the olive oil in a dutch oven over medium heat. Add the onion, celery, and carrots and cook, stirring occasionally, for 5 minutes until lightly browned. Add the mushrooms and sauté for 2 minutes. Add the garlic, thyme, and oregano and cook, stirring, for 2 minutes.

4. Add the broth, wild rice, 1½ teaspoons of the kosher salt, and the pepper. Bring the soup to a simmer. Simmer uncovered for 20 minutes, then add the beans and continue to simmer, uncovered, for 30–35 minutes more, or until the rice breaks open.

5. Using a liquid cup measure, carefully remove 2 cups of the hot soup (including broth, veggies, and rice) to a blender. Add 1 cup water. Drain the cashews and add them to the soup in the blender along with the dried sage. Blend on high for about 1 minute until smooth, then pour the mixture back into the soup.

6. Add the soy sauce and the remaining ½ teaspoon kosher salt. Taste and adjust seasoning as desired. Garnish with fresh ground pepper.

KIMBERLY'S IMMUNE-BOOSTING SHAKES

One of the very best things you can do for your health is to have a smoothie for breakfast every day. A smoothie with the right combination of green leafy vegetables and fruits packed with vitamins, minerals, and antioxidants is the single best way to reduce inflammation generally in your body and to recover from a workout.

Any form of exercise causes stress to your body, which you then need to heal from. Obviously, the goal is for your body to adapt to the stress you've placed on it, thereby getting stronger/faster/better before the next workout.

Boost your nutrition with microgreens. Microgreens are a great way to add nutrients to any meal or smoothie. Nutritious microgreens include wheatgrass, watercress, alfalfa sprouts, sunflower sprouts, pea sprouts, clover sprouts, and lentil sprouts.

5D Green Anti-Inflammatory Smoothie

INGREDIENTS:

2 large kale leaves (stems removed and discarded)
1 large handful of spinach
1 frozen or fresh banana
1 cup frozen or fresh blueberries
1 cup frozen or fresh blackberries
1 cup frozen or fresh mango
2 cups water or nondairy milk (almond milk or oat milk or flaxseed milk)
1 tablespoon hemp hearts
1 tablespoon flaxseed
¼ teaspoon ground ginger (Having a positive attitude and using the best possible quality ingredients available, I substitute ginger for turmeric.)

DIRECTIONS:

Place all the ingredients in a high-speed blender and blend on high for 1 minute or until desired consistency. Happy Health!

Kimberly's 5D Immune Booster Smoothie

This yummy smoothie is perfect for a healthy snack that also rebuilds the immune system!

In a blender, combine the following ingredients:

2 cups liquid, any combination of:
Spring water
Coconut water
Almond milk
Flaxseed milk

Add 2 cups fruit, any combination of:
Goji berries
Blueberries
Blackberries
Pear
Apple
Mango

Add 1 cup tightly packed dark leafy greens, such as:
Spinach
Kale
Romaine
Watercress
Microgreens
Beet greens
Collard greens

Add ½ cup hemp protein powder
Add 2 teaspoons freshly grated ginger
Add 4 mint leaves

Blend well and enjoy!

The Peachy Pear Smoothie

INGREDIENTS:
   ½ small apple, sliced
   1 peach, sliced
   1 pear, sliced
   Juice of ½ lemon
   ¾ inch fresh ginger, peeled
   1 cup unsweetened almond or cashew milk
   1 scoop soy-free protein powder (optional)
   1 tablespoon chia seeds
   3 handfuls microgreens like watercress

DIRECTIONS:

Blend all the ingredients in a blender until smooth.

Cancer-Fighting Smoothie

If you're looking for a cancer-fighting smoothie, then you need this recipe. My anti-cancer green breakfast smoothie is dairy-free and vegan, with frozen or fresh organic broccoli and other ingredients that have been shown to help fight diseases, including cancer.

INGREDIENTS:

¼ cup hemp seeds
3 cups filtered spring water
1 cup frozen mango or sweet cherries
¼ cup frozen or fresh pomegranate arils
1 1-inch knob fresh ginger
2 cups fresh salad greens or lightly steamed kale, spinach, or collard greens
10 fresh mint leaves
2 tablespoons cocoa powder
1 cup frozen raw broccoli florets
juice of one lime

DIRECTIONS:

Place all the ingredients in a blender and process until smooth.

You may have this smoothie to boost your immune system at least three times a week, in addition to wheatgrass juice three times a week. It can also be used as a cancer preventative.

Kimberly's 5D Smoothie Shake

To strengthen your immune system, try my delicious smoothie drink recipe custom-made for immunosuppressed individuals.

In a blender, combine the following ingredients:
2 cups liquid, any combination of:
Spring water
Coconut water
Almond milk
Flaxseed milk

Add 2 cups fruit, any combination of:
Goji berries
Blueberries
Blackberries
Pear
Apple
Mango

Add 1 cup tightly packed dark leafy greens, such as:
Spinach
Kale
Romaine
Watercress
Microgreens
Beet greens
Collard greens
Spirulina (Limit spinach and spirulina to no more than twice a week.)

Add ½ cup hemp protein powder
Add 2 teaspoons freshly grated ginger
Add 4 mint leaves

Blend well and enjoy!

5D TEETH AND GUM CARE

Many of my clients' immune systems are under attack due to bacterial infections, which often begin in the gums and teeth and travel to the lymph nodes. The latest scientific research suggests a connection between poor oral health, such as chronic periodontal or gum disease, and several chronic diseases, including diabetes, heart disease, stroke, Alzheimer's, and certain cancers.

What is the secret to teeth and gum care? Correct brushing and flossing, knowing which foods and drinks to eat and which to avoid, and having regular dental checkups can all help keep your teeth and gums healthy, your smile beautiful, and your mouth free from infections and bad breath. I am a true believer that good health begins with good dental care and good drinking water.

Fluoride and Health

For several decades, increasing numbers of municipalities throughout the United States have been fluoridating their water, ostensibly for the purposes of reducing the rate of tooth decay. However, most of Western Europe does not have fluoridated water, yet their rate of tooth decay is no higher than in the United States.

There is also evidence that fluoride can pose various health risks. Fluoride can cause harm to proteins in soft tissues, including the blood, brain, and liver, where it can penetrate cellular membranes. Some scientific research has also linked fluoride with lower IQ in children. Various groups have raised additional concerns that fluoride may be associated with a number of other diseases and health conditions.

There is also a concern of over-fluoridation, where people are exposed to too much fluoride. Because fluoride is present in so many products, in addition to water and toothpaste, it can be very easy for an individual to be exposed to far more fluoride than is necessary, even for the purpose of cavity reduction.

Because both fluoride and aluminum can pass through the blood-brain barrier—the structure that protects the brain from toxins—an additional concern arises for those who have fluoridated water and who cook in aluminum pots. There is a possibility that the fluoride in the water can combine with the aluminum in the pot and form aluminum fluoride. Aluminum and aluminum fluoride can combine with oxygen to form aluminum oxide, a compound found in the brains of Alzheimer's patients, and is also associated with osteoporosis, osteomalacia, spontaneous bone fractures, and dementia.

For those who have fluoridated water, I recommend cooking with—and drinking—quality spring water. I recommend cooking with glass or stainless steel. I do not recommend cooking with aluminum or Teflon.

For those who are interested in fluoride for cavity prevention, consider alternative toothpastes that contain a new generation of materials that can replace lost tooth enamel. For example, Apagard toothpaste from Japan contains a special form of hydroxyapatite—the material that comprises tooth enamel—to rebuild tooth enamel in those at risk of, or experiencing, tooth decay.

THE 5D LIST OF HEALTH DOS AND DON'TS

What to Embrace:

- Taking a multivitamin
- Taking certain supplements, if they are right for you
- Taking probiotics
- Getting exercise
- Having a spiritual practice
- Meditating
- Enjoying music
- Performing service work or giving back to the community in some way
- Eating healthy fruits and vegetables
- Getting enough sleep
- Minimizing stress
- Drinking spring water—but not out of plastic bottles

- Bathing using a Rainshower bath ball or showering with water run through a Rainshower dechlorinating filter
- Eating organic food
- Using an EMF meter, checking the areas of your home, where you spend the most time, for excessive electromagnetic radiation, giving special attention to areas where people sleep

What to Avoid

- Exposure to electromagnetic radiation from microwave ovens, cell phones by your head and bed at night, Wi-Fi routers, wireless devices, including Bluetooth and wireless headsets, and so on; also try to reduce exposure to power line and cell phone tower radiation.
- Plastics, especially when eating and drinking (plastics leach toxic chemicals into whatever food or drink they contain)
- Drinking or bathing in unfiltered tap water
- Drinking from refrigerator water filters and from well water
- Smoking
- Eating fish
- Drinking alcohol in excess
- Consuming soy
- Consuming genetically modified ingredients
- Chemical cleaners and pollutants

- Using butane when cooking (the fumes are toxic)
- Exposure to synthetic chemicals as much as possible
- Dyes, soaps, and chemicals for hair or clothes
- Fluorescent lighting
- Standard LED screens

SIMPLE WAYS TO PROTECT YOUR EYES, YOUR MOOD, AND YOUR SLEEP QUALITY

- Use OLED lighting for your home and at work if possible. This is organic light-emitting diode; it reduces power consumption and is better on your eyes.
- Choose bulbs that emit orange and yellow hues to reduce your exposure to blue light. You may have to try different shades to find one that you like. The right shade of yellow or orange can reduce anxiety, reduce insomnia, and improve sleep. Blue light destroys melatonin and contributes to anxiety and insomnia. All white light bulbs emit blue light.
- Wear yellow or orange sunglasses that block light in the blue spectrum as well as all forms of UV radiation. One such brand is Swanwick's Night Swannies. These are especially helpful when you need to go to a place that has harsh lighting, such as is often found at typical grocery or department

stores, schools or universities, hospitals, or government buildings. The Guides hope that the world will have OLED in all essentials soon.

- Use device features to reduce blue light emitted from electronic screens. On Windows, this feature is called Night Light. On a Mac, this feature is called Night Shift. You can also use a program called f.lux.

- You can install apps that reduce blue light on your cell phone and tablet screens. Such apps are available in various app stores. Just be sure you choose a highly rated app that also respects and protects your privacy.

EPILOGUE

My wish for you, as you experience holding and reading this book, is that you let go of any fear emanating from the lower self and that you fill yourself with only love as you travel, journey, and voyage with your Guides and me into the 5th Dimension.

I see the world differently from most people. I experience the 5th Dimension daily, which is like living inside a spiritual glass menagerie. My eyes see through a colorful kaleidoscopic world guided by a nonjudgmental God Frequency who loves all.

My wish for you is that you feel excited about the life you want to live, that you find your gifts, and that you enhance your abilities in the 5th Dimension. I am so blessed and happy to serve you on these pages. I came from so far away to reach you. I love you. My Guides are kind and active in communication with your Guides.

I'll feel blessed and utterly grateful if you have even one moment of awe, of reverence of life—your life!—during the turning of any of these pages. I hope you come to experience the excitement of knowing that through suffering, pain, and dying, we are given a rebirth, and we can live many lives inside of one life.

For example, I have had multiple NDEs, through which I

became who I am. Reading this book, you may discover you have also had an NDE.

How I live my days here on Earth is by walking my own path. My wish for you is to overcome any hardships with the highest strength. By living in the 5th Dimensional Godliness, it's an easier journey to voyage embracing the destination to enlightenment.

When I first met Dr. C. Norman Shealy for a scientific testing of my abilities, I had to fly out to Missouri. It was a big journey. I didn't know what to expect. I was to be tested on eighteen individuals who served as patient test subjects. Dr. Shealy was very strict. This was an intense experience, but I knew this was what God wanted. As the patients received my medical intuitive readings and healings, Dr. Shealy watched with his lovely grin as he recorded results and took many notations. My Guides found cancer, tumors, torn knee injuries, and so on. One test subject had a large, hard lymph node on the left side of her neck.

"This is not good," I said.

"I have to have it surgically removed," she replied.

Dr. Shealy got up from his desk, walked over and touched the node with his index finger, looked at me with his blue eyes, and said, "Yes, it sure is there."

"Let's pray together," I said.

"What do you mean?" she asked.

"If we pray," I replied, "I will place my hands on your node, enter the 5th Dimension, and release the node off your neck through the Holy Spirit. If you believe, you shall be healed."

She wanted to say the Hail Mary prayer, and Dr. Shealy

and I recited the prayer with her. The node dissolved out of my hands and off her neck. Dr. Shealy placed his index finger to the side of her neck; he looked back up at me and said, "It's gone." I will never forget his look! I was so happy, and my body was chilled. We all honored God. The woman placed her hand on her neck and was extremely grateful and also taken by the experience, but being spiritual, she was not surprised. Dr. Shealy said to me, "The power of God is using you as an agent."

"Well," I said to them, "we can all be used by God in this way."

I felt at that time that I was just starting to see the power of the Holy Spirit. Since then, I have seen multiple tumors dissolve in two minutes out of my hands, just as I had been healed many times. My eyes have seen suffering and pain since I was a very small child. I also have seen many Miracles.

The 5th Dimension is here to help you find your blessings, find the breath you came into the world with, and to help you to connect to your heart consciousness and your gifts of the Holy Spirit.

Know that you are multidimensional, just as this book is multidimensional. The fact that you are reading this book is an absolute honor to me. Please know this is true. Everyone and everything is energy. And so is this book you're reading.

The Holy Divine energy is real and here to help us say, "No fear!" It's here to help us to say "Yes!" to love, to never have a doubt, to have unmovable faith because the Omnipresent and All is miraculous!

That I'm even here to channel these words to you as a soul being reborn many times, as the observer, amazes me and fills me with gratitude and overwhelming joy. I now know how much you universally matter to the Guides.

You learn and grow to serve. Awaken to the fact that it is possible for you to say, "I am alive in this time in history where Christ light is one and I am awakened and aligned with the Universal Being, healed with all. I am one with God."

I can have the power within me to matter, to reach my higher universal consciousness. I can use my love for my brothers and sisters and have peace inside my soul. This is the most important, magical, exciting time to flow with the positive and dismiss any negative. When you are in the 5th Dimension, your consciousness believes in the Holy Spirit, which is universal love.

Let this be the beginning of your new life in the 5th Dimension—the Dimension of the Spirit.

Channeled by Kimberly Meredith

APPENDIX 1

5th Dimension Resources

HEALING PRODUCTS I RECOMMEND

In all cases, use as directed, and also in cooperation with your health care practitioner. (Unless otherwise indicated, I am not compensated for recommending these products.)

Healthy Supplements

- *Solgar multivitamins*—including the following (available at online retailers; *I do not profit from their sale*): B6, B3, and B12: 100 mg veggie caps, vitamin C, D3 5,000 IU (take as directed), selenium 200 mcg/day, lysine 1,500 mg/day, GABA (for anxiety), zinc.

- *Testa*—Fish-free algae-based Omega Acid EPA & DHA

- *David Wolfe's Coated Silver*—99.99 percent bioavailable colloidal silver. I am an affiliate, and I use this product and love it. Go to www.thehealingtrilogy.com/store.

- *Dr. Norm Shealy's Biogenics*—Magnesium Lotion and Magnesium Lotion Spray. Apply as directed. See www.normshealy.com.

- *U-Tract Complete* by Progressive Laboratories (for urinary tract)—Take as directed on the bottle. Available at many online retailers.

- *G5 Siliplant* (oral liquid)—Take as directed on the bottle. Available at many online retailers.

- *Silicium G5 gel* (external use for joints)—Take as directed on the bottle. Available at many online retailers.

- *Inner-ēco coconut probiotic (plain)*—(for digestive health)—Available at Whole Foods or Sprouts.

Healthy Water Products

- *Rainshower Bath Ball*—See www.rainshower.com.

- *Rainshower CQ-1000-NH dechlorinating shower*—See www.rainshower.com.

- *Mountain Valley spring water*—See www.mountainvalleyspring.com.

Healthy Consumer Products

- *Tom's of Maine*—Toothpaste without fluoride. Available at many retail outlets.

- *OLED light bulbs*—These emit a softer, diffuse, glare-free light that is healthier for the eyes. Available at retail outlets.

- *Swanwick's Night Swannies sunglasses*—See www.swanwicksleep.com.

- *AIR Doctor Purifier*—The first affordable air purifier that not only removes almost 100 percent of particles but also the vast majority of toxic ozone, volatile organic chemicals, and gases. I am an affiliate, and I use this product and love it. Go to www.thehealingtrilogy.com/store.

- *Ozonated water*—Can be made at home with an ozone machine and a bubbler. Ozonate water for ten to twenty minutes. Consume within ten minutes, as the ozone will dissipate quickly. These machines are available online starting around fifty dollars.

- *Hyperbaric oxygen therapy*—Requires a doctor's prescription. Hyperbaric oxygen therapy is a well-established treatment for serious infections, head injuries, immunosuppressed conditions, bubbles of air in your blood vessels, and wounds that won't heal as a result of diabetes or radiation injury. Can be purchased online for home therapy.

- *Margaret McCormick*—Soul removal and aura-healing practitioner. I highly recommend her for spiritual cleansing. See www.margaretmccormick.com.

My Products from My Online Store, *www.thehealingtrilogy .com/store*

- *Angel Awakening* Album
  - Guided Healing Meditations
  - Written and spoken word by Kimberly Meredith
  - Angelic music by Steven Halpern
  - A voyage through the Angelic Realm to discover your own healing, with uplifting lyrics written by Kimberly and Angelic music by Grammy-nominated composer Steven Halpern, widely regarded as one of the founding fathers of new age music. Steven Halpern also produced the album. The Angels are here to help you awaken to the best version of yourself.

- *Kimberly Meredith Channels the Holy Spirit Meditation Healing* CD
  - Kimberly's CD release takes you on an ocean ride into surrendering yourself to the higher self of love and light . . . out of 3rd Dimensional pain, worry, and fear . . . and into the 5th Dimensional higher cosmic consciousness. Calling for global peace and healing, for body, mind, and Spirit, Kimberly channeled this entire recording through Holy Spirit and many masters.

Relax and breathe it in. God is here. This album was engineered by Grammy-winning producer Matt Wallace. See www .thehealingtrilogy.com/store/. It can also be purchased from iTunes and CDBaby.com and listened to on Pandora.

- Blessed Ormus Cream

  - My exclusive line of Blessed Ormus Cream has been personally prayed over by me, infused with God's Healing Energy, and confirmed by my Guides as beneficial. Ormus is known to help communication between the body and Spirit as well as between the cells. I have experienced natural healing and wellness through this organic alchemy that comes from the sea.

    Ormus cream can help activate the third eye, throat chakra, and DNA, including the twelve interdimensional layers of energy that surround DNA. It increases mental focus, clarity, sense of calmness, rejuvenation, and intuition. Most people have also reported a remarkable improvement in vision, a decrease of menopausal symptoms, and better digestion.

    Long-term ingestion produces cellular life, lengthens telomeres, and reverses aging, improving cellular structuring and rejuvenation. It has the capacity to activate cellular enzymes.

    Ingredients: 100 percent organic: oils, plant-based wax, Dead Sea salt minerals, human resonance (HR) Ormus, colloidal silver. Oils used: sunflower, olive, grape seed, castor oil, coconut oil.

    (I am an affiliate, and I use this product and love it.)

- *AIR Doctor Purifier*—see page 216 for more information.

- *David Wolfe's Coated Silver*—99.99 percent bioavailable colloidal silver. I am an affiliate, and I use this product and love it. Go to: www.thehealingtrilogy.com/store.

SCIENCE RESOURCES TO PROTECT YOUR HEALTH FROM EXPOSURE TO PLASTICS

- *Ecology Center:* Adverse Health Effects of Plastics—https://ecologycenter.org/factsheets/adverse-health-effects-of-plastics/.

- *Consumer Reports:* How to Eat Less Plastic—https://www.consumerreports.org/food/how-to-eat-less-plastic-microplastics-in-food-water/.

- *Environmental Health News:* Plastic Threatens Our Health—https://www.ehn.org/plastic-pollution-and-human-health-2629322391.html.

- *Plastic Pollution Coalition:* Report: Plastic Threatens Human Health—https://www.plasticpollutioncoalition.org/blog/2019/2/20/report-plastic-threatens-human-health-at-a-global-scale.

MY BOOK SUGGESTIONS

- Paramahansa Yogananda, *Autobiography of a Yogi* and *Whispers from Eternity.*

- C. Norman Shealy, M.D., Ph.D. *Conversations with G: A Physician's Encounter with Heaven.*

- Wayne W. Dyer, *The Shift: Taking Your Life from Ambition to Meaning* and *Memories of Heaven.*

- Eckhart Tolle, *The Power of Now.*

- Richard Bach, *Illusions: The Adventures of a Reluctant Messiah.*

- Rainer Maria Rilke, *Letters to a Young Poet.*

- The Dalai Lama and Desmond Tutu, *The Book of Joy: Lasting Happiness in a Changing World.*

- Paul Selig, *I Am the Word: A Guide to the Consciousness of Man's Self in a Transitioning Time.*

- Bruce Fife, N.D., and Conrado Dayrit, *Coconut Cures: Preventing and Treating Common Health Problems with Coconut.*

- Thomas John, *Never Argue with a Dead Person.*

APPENDIX 2

Kimberly's Stories of Miraculous Healings

Following are stories of people I worked with and their experiences of healing. While these are stories of people who worked with me directly, my hope is that these stories inspire you to explore all the 5th Dimension teachings in this book, do the practices, and begin your own healing journey.

COLON CANCER MIRACLE HEALINGS

One of our 9/11 heroes, a New York City policeman who saved many lives at the Twin Towers, came to my office in Los Angeles, accompanied by his girlfriend. He introduced himself to me. "I am Bob, and I have heard you are very good at finding things with your mediumship, and I heard you work with the Holy Spirit. Whatever you say, I will do. I am a believer. I have children and grandkids, and I want to live."

I felt chills when he said that. He had been a New York City police officer for over a decade and prior to that had been in the U.S. Marines. He said he had something going on in his body, but he wouldn't tell me what it was. He lay down, and his girlfriend sat in a chair next to him. They both looked very sad. As I got ready to scan him, he asked if he could tape record the session, and I said, "Absolutely, you can record it," which I always recommend because my Guides give so much detailed information, so fast, that recordings are advisable.

While I scanned him, I waved my right hand over his body and got guided information, in sync with coded eye blinking, in different multidimensional codes. I guided him into a 5th Dimensional energy. I knew instantly he had cancer because I was getting hot flashes, and my right eye was blinking faster.

I felt the Holy Spirit go through my body, and then I started counting the tumors. I counted sixteen of them, but the main one, the most dangerous one, was attached to his colon. When I detect cancer in someone, hot flashes go through my body. My left eye blinks "yes" when something is good, and my right eye blinks "no" if there is something going on that isn't good. Anytime I find a tumor, my right eye blinks.

When I told him what I found, he confirmed it. "You're right. I have Stage IV colon cancer. And it's metastasized."

I asked him to hold selenite crystals in his hands to ground his energy. (These crystals are high-vibration stones that absorb negative energies and balance the chakras when held.) He was very open and ready for his healing. He kept saying over and over, "I know God can heal me." When I laid my hands on the area of the cancerous tumor, my eyes were blinking on where to guide my hands, and I asked him to pray with me. He opened his hands, and he started to shiver and the crystals dropped from his hands. When that happened, the Holy Spirit went right through his body. He kept praying the Hail Mary over and over again. He said he felt a tingling sensation going through his body. As I was praying on him, my hands were numb and my lips were tingling and I felt the Spirit of the Divine telling me that he would be healed. I held back my tears from knowing he would be healed.

Mother Mary's energy had come into the room. This man was a very spiritual man, and he was in all the way, as a complete believer in this process. He began sobbing. He felt guilty that when he went into one of the Twin Towers for the last time, to pull people out, he had been unable to save a firefighter who was one of his friends. Bob had come out holding the body of a dead girl, and he was so devastated; he thought that absorbing this traumatic energy and the resulting guilt was why he got cancer.

We released that negative energy out through the prayer of Mother Mary, and he felt relief that first day from the work we did together. Though he had many tumors, I continued to feel the most significant one to be on his colon, and I went right to it with my healing hands. He recoiled in pain. "Owwwww!" I started pushing on it and started moving it around while saying, "Hail Mary, Hail Mary." We prayed and prayed together.

That night, after Bob left my office, he was rushed to the hospital. Because of the way the tumor on his colon had previously been positioned, they hadn't been able to surgically remove it. But because of our prayer and how I moved the tumor through the Holy Spirit, it shifted through my hands-on surgery. His doctors were then able to easily cut the tumor out of him, which they hadn't been able to do until the tumor was moved during our healing session.

Here is something he wrote in his daily journal: "I am fighting cancer again today and need another surgery, but it's all good. I'm keeping up with my chemo and the help of Kimberly Meredith's spiritual guidance and her helping me boost my immune system with her nutritional program and the energy of God's prayers. We read life is short and many times it doesn't move as fast as we like but if the end of the tunnel of light turns out to be a train better to gain an appreciation of life that we never had or the train will run you down. Life is beautiful. Another six rounds. I'm not going to stop. I'm going for it."

For my clients who battle cancer, going through chemo and radiation can be so difficult. With chemo, you don't have sensation in your hands anymore, you're numb, you have neuropathy, and you've lost your appetite. You can't drive a car anymore. Bob was the rare exception among my clients because he had cancer everywhere in most of his internal organs.

When I am scanning, I feel the energy field, and I can tell if someone is going to live or not. I know instantly if that person is going to fight it and win, or give up the fight. I had a feeling that Bob was on the cusp, to be honest. I wasn't sure he would make it for two reasons. One, he felt very beaten down. He was a big, strong guy on the outside, but experienced post-traumatic stress and was traumatized emotionally. He was so sensitive that even going to his chemo and radiation, he was feeling for everyone else in there going through chemo and radiation. Bob was also on a lot of painkillers.

I thought there was a point where he was giving up. Then, all of a sudden, he shifted and became extremely strong and even more dedicated. It was on the day when he came into the office and I had to give him tough love. I looked into his eyes, and we had a spiritual counseling session and he told me how sad he was seeing so many of his cancer peers dying. He was telling them he had been seeing me and that he was healed.

I expressed to him how he was here as a conduit for his healing and to be of service to others after this whole journey was over, but everyone is responsible for their own healing journey. He said he had always been of service in his life and now he feels his life will lead to being of service to God. He understood he had to go through this experience, and after that, I saw a shift in him. He even stopped taking painkillers.

I saw a reflection of myself through Bob when I had been on my painkillers for over a year, and I knew how hard it was to release the painkillers to receive the biggest gift of the Holy Spirit. Bob will tell you personally that he had to give up the oxycodone and all the painkillers to become closer to God and go back to being the fighter he was during 9/11. He had numbed out the pain through medication, which was exactly what I had done a few years earlier.

A lot of people with cancer and serious diseases sometimes become reliant on painkillers, and therefore they get extremely depressed, which suppresses their immune system. There are less harmful alternatives to take the pain away, such as oxygen therapy and sound healing (see the resource appendix). We feel we need painkillers for pain relief, of course, and sometimes we do, but to become reliant on them for too long can only lead us to become immunosuppressed.

He finally went cold off them and was grateful. He decided to start exercising and get more intimately involved with his family.

He had six more rounds of chemo and numerous surgeries. Once he threw the painkillers into the toilet, it brought more connection to the Omnipresent in his body. He continued to see me weekly with me praying over him and his continued program. Any time he would get bad news about his prognosis, he would say, "I am healed." 5D healing keeps us focused on our healing, rather than on our fear.

This had been a dead man walking with metastasized colon cancer, so it was nothing short of miraculous the transformation he underwent.

I gave him a nutritional supplement plan that involved using inner-ēco (a probiotic) and vitamins, supplements, and an organic nutritional program, along with lifestyle changes, as you found outlined earlier. It was a homework plan, which made him happy. He went home and did everything on it.

He texted me: "They told me I had advanced stage four colon cancer and they gave me between six weeks and three months to live, which obviously isn't pleasant to hear. And now after nine surgeries, and thirty-eight rounds (or doses) of chemotherapy, and three rounds of radiation, my cancer markers are down to normal and my blood is all good. Cancer has changed me forever. Thank you, Kimberly."

He wrote:

People ask me how do you get rid of or tolerate all of that pain. I don't do anything but allow myself to feel it. The body shifts energy for survival. Once you understand that, you make pain your friend, so that it teaches you a lesson rather than hurts you. Then you just grow and live your best life. Pain is a necessary inconvenience to inner peace. Thank you for coming into my life weekly to guide me through this crazy cancer battle. I am grateful for Kimberly Meredith for her healing energy and laying hands on me, for enlightening me and opening me up to spirituality, for healing me.

Some clients are running scared and scatter themselves every-where, trying every type of vitamin and a lot of different healers. He stayed focused working with me and stayed in his heart and trusted my Spirit Guides. He also worked with his oncologist and he asked my Guides which chemo therapy would work best for him. People do that all the time with me. They stay healed by keeping their immune system strong, eating healthfully, and by maintaining their spiritual practice. You cannot live the lifestyle you had before you got sick.

Our firefighters and police officers are heroes, and when they and the nurses and doctors needing help come in to see me, they are all so honorable, so in the Spirit, and so very ready to be healed. They are open channels for healing so they can go back out there and be of service to others.

A CHILD MIRACLE HEALING

Marisa came to my office after her mother heard about me from a man who had prostate cancer, who had been healed. Marisa was born with GI tract issues and had never had normal bowel movements. She had just turned four when I saw her, and she wanted to sit on my lap as soon as she arrived. She had been to see lots of doctors and tried lots of diets and medications. She had blood in her stool and had been vomiting for several days, and she was very underweight and in pain that day. She was a candidate for developing cancer because her im-mune system was so compromised.

She grabbed the two white crystals I do healing with, wanting me to put the holy water on her. She got up on the table and asked me to heal her. I started to scan her without knowing she had gastrointesti-nal issues. Her mother, Terri, had only said her daughter was sick. I immediately went to her lower intestinal tract and felt she was having pain there. I also felt a lot of emotion in Marisa; she was very sad because she wasn't able to do what her nursery school classmates did.

As I did the healing work, she was praying, and because she is from a Catholic family, she knew the Haily Mary prayer. She opened her hands up and breathed very hard. Her grandmother and mom were nearby, also praying and saying a lot of Hail Marys. I kept hearing my Guides say her intestines were out of place, and I tried to move them back into place. I pushed down on her esophagus and into her intestinal tract. The Guides were doing psychic surgery on her. She was so unbelievably relaxed, in the 5th Dimensional frequency, and she kept chanting and praying and wanting to be healed.

She got in my lap and kissed me when we finished and said, "I am healed." And I said back to her, "Yes, you are healed."

Later, I got an email from her mother, who said when they got in the car after our session, Marisa vomited, but the next day, she could eat and drink normally and she was having regular bowel movements. One month later, her whole intestinal tract was completely healed, and she hasn't had a problem since. Marisa said that God put her intestinal tract back through the Holy Spirit, and her doctor confirmed that she's been totally healed.

Terri wrote to me:

Hi my name is Terri, and my daughter is Marisa, who just turned five. She was born with gastro-intestinal problems. She would wake up two to three times a night in pain crying that her tummy hurt. She had been seeing a specialist for a few years and they had done an endoscopy on her, and an upper GI on her, and they determined that it was gastritis. She was taking about a dozen or so different types of medications and nothing had helped. One day one of my co-workers told me about Kimberly. So I made an appointment to bring my daughter in and see Kimberly. That day Kimberly did surgery, through her surgical hands. God healed my daughter, and now she is doing wonderful. She's eating and she's a happy child. I'm just very glad I came.

I am happy to say I saw Marisa six months later and she was back at school, taking my protocol diet plan, chanting the prayers with my CD, and she has never had any of the symptoms since she had a healing with me that day.

BREAST CANCER MIRACLES

I met Christy through a Skype session she signed up for after she heard about me on YouTube. She was a thirty-five-year-old owner of a hair salon, going through relationship stress. Though she didn't live very far from me, she was too busy with her salon to come in person, so she made a Skype appointment.

She never told me anything was physically wrong with her. She mainly wanted to talk about her emotional turmoil and issues with her boyfriend, which involved me giving her spiritual counseling. As I did this, I started to get instant hot flashes and a download from a Spirit Guide. I began doing my medical Medium scan on her with a wave of my right hand across her body. I kept focusing on her chest and getting hot flashes, which I get when I am cued in on something. We did a full-body scan using the computer screen, and I waved my hand across the screen looking at her body, and I kept blinking on her left breast where I felt a dark energy. At that moment, I knew it was cancer, though she didn't know.

I told Christy she needed more love in her life, which made her cry. I suggested she get her breast checked out with her doctor and get a mammogram. She was shocked because she didn't feel anything in her breast. She kept saying she had no symptoms at all. But she did everything I suggested, and I put her on vitamins and probiotics because I sensed she had a weak immune system.

She did say she would see her gynecologist, and I didn't hear from her for about three weeks. Then she booked an appointment with me in person and came into my office looking concerned but happy. She explained how she had told her doctor that she had a scan with a Medium. When she said that, I had chills and hot flashes that she had cancer. She started to cry.

"I have Stage I breast cancer, and you caught it early," she said.

"I wouldn't have known if I hadn't had the session with you. Praise God."

When I did a scan over her, where they did the biopsy, I laid my hand on her left breast and felt the lump. She opened up her hands and went into the 5th Dimension, using her breath, inhaling through her nose and exhaling through her mouth. I started to pray. She repeated, "I am love, and I am light. And I am healed."

As I put my hand on the lump, I felt it diminishing in size, and so did she. I prayed to Mother Mary, and we did a lot of forgiveness prayers together to break a cord of negative energy over her from her mother and her boyfriend. We also did oxygen therapy and aroma-therapy, using mint, lemon, and eucalyptus.

Christy later emailed me this testimonial:

I had a medical medium scan on Skype with Kimberly. She went right to the lump in my left breast. She suggested getting a mammogram and I did have a mammogram and ultrasound, which found the lump had all the characteristics of cancer. Then I had a biopsy and was diagnosed with stage one cancer. Kimberly found it first, in its early stage, so I was able to catch it early because of her. My doctor said to me this is the best example of early detection of breast cancer. I'm really glad I did that, before I was getting symptoms, and before it spread to my breast tissue.

She had an early stage of invasive breast cancer, and it was two centimeters and no lymph nodes were involved. When I laid hands on it, it shrank to one centimeter. She still had to have a lumpectomy to cut it out, and she did five days of radiation for five weeks as an outpatient.

As a result of the Miracle healing, she made decisions to eliminate negative people from her life who depleted her energy field, and the experience brought her closer to God.

SALLY'S BREAST CANCER MIRACLE

Another breast cancer client of mine, Sally, in her sixties, had something called a one-centimeter invasive lobular carcinoma. She came
into my office after she had already been diagnosed but didn't tell me
of her diagnosis. She was upset with her diagnosis and wanted me to
scan her. I did a routine scan because she was confused about what
direction she wanted to go with her treatment. Her doctors wanted to
do a lumpectomy. As I proceeded to do the scan on her, I waved my
hand straight to her right breast and directly to her uterus; my right
eye blinked on both these areas, and on her thyroid and the back of
her neck, the T1 area.

"When is the last time you had your hormones checked?" I asked
her. And she started to cry. She said her oncologist was convinced that
she had gotten the invasive lobular carcinoma from being on high
doses of prescription estrogen for thirteen years, after having had a
previous hysterectomy. She wished she had gone the holistic route for
hormonal therapy instead of taking pharmaceutical estrogen.

She asked me to do a healing on her, and I guided her into the
5th Dimension. I asked her to breathe in through her nose and exhale
through her mouth as she held on to the selenite crystals. She commented that she felt the energy of Mother Mary go through her body.
She cried through the healing and felt a beautiful release and healing through Mother Mary. She was already eating healthy, but I suggested she begin using probiotics, as well as drinking Mountain Valley
spring water that was ozonated, as well as wheatgrass juice. I spiritually helped to move her into understanding that she needed to also allow Western medicine to help her by doing the lumpectomy to release
some nodes that needed to be taken out. I was successful in shrinking
down the mass, but she still needed to have the procedure done.

She wrote me two weeks later, after her procedure:

Praise God AND Mother Mary, who was with me every breath
of the way! It was all easy, just like you and the Guides prayed
it would be. I am SO very grateful! Surgeon just called with

pathology results. Excellent news!! NO CANCER anywhere! Margins are clear, lymph nodes are clear; tumor completely removed. SO grateful!!!!! Best news ever!!! The Doctors even were so amazed! Thank you for all your support and love!

JANE'S BREAST CANCER MIRACLE

Everyone has a different outcome with the Divine and how their healing turns out. You can never go wrong with prayer and alternative care. In the case of Jane, she came into my office wanting a scan. She had been to a prominent breast surgeon in Beverly Hills who wanted to remove a benign breast tumor, but she was adamant about not wanting it surgically removed.

She was in her thirties, of Jewish faith, and had just come from her breast surgeon's office. She told me she had a mass in her breast that probably needed to be removed, and she asked me to take a look. She had heard of me and my work, and she also wanted to get closer to the energy of God.

I began to scan her, and the energy of the Divine found the lump in her breast. I looked into her eyes and asked her to accept the Holy Spirit. She said she would accept the Spirit and breathed and prayed with me, and we released the negative energy from her breast. I took her hand and had her feel where the lump had been, and she was shocked and happy that it was gone. We put our hands up in the air and said, "Praise God, Hashem, Hashem." (*Hashem* is Hebrew for God.) After every healing, we should praise God in this manner.

She came back for a second session and brought her ultrasound images of her breast showing the mass was gone.

Jane later wrote to me:

Working with Kimberly has changed my life in the most magnificent ways. Her hands on healing removed a benign tumor in three minutes that had been in my right breast for 20 years.

The top, prominent surgeon was flabbergasted after two confirmation visits and she printed ultrasound photos to show me. Kimberly's love, healing, guidance and communion with the Holy Spirit as The Healing Trilogy has opened my world up in the most amazing, joyful, magical ways. I am forever grateful and my faith in our God is unquestionable and continues to get stronger. I am beyond grateful to have met her and connected to this energy.

People have been healed by my voice on the radio, listening to my CDs, and while watching my videos.

HEART DISEASE HEALED

A client of mine, Sean, works as a movie actor and comes from a family of doctors, but he believes in holistic healing. He heard about me through referrals. As I performed a routine medical intuitive scan across his body with my hands and my eyes, I began to receive negative blinks focused around his heart area. He confirmed that he had a heart condition, and he was very concerned about it because it could affect his ability to perform as a pro surfer. I also found additional injuries that had happened to him, such as on his left knee from when he had a surfing accident.

He asked me to do a laying on of hands around his heart area. He truly wanted to gain more of a connection to the Divine. As I did the healing on him, I felt he truly was accepting and receiving of the energy of the Divine. Usually the condition, which involves a heart valve that doesn't close tightly, is fixed surgically.

After the first treatment, I saw a significant difference in him. The doctors also agreed after his stress test they saw a positive outcome. I recommended he walk around his neighborhood three times a week, and surf again in about a month and eat a low saturated non trans-fat diet, low in sugar and salt. His cardio-echo stress test results miraculously improved, and he no longer had the symptoms he had been experiencing.

Two years after treatment, he remains significantly improved and his doctors have given him a complete thumbs-up.

Sean wrote to me:

> I had my echo stress test and passed with flying colors, the heart looks great, the doctor said, you have a happy heart, this is incredible. It's odd that at peak performance I am testing like a professional athlete. For some odd reason there is less heart regurgitation. I don't understand. This is an absolute miracle. The mitral valve is functioning beyond great. This is an amazing miracle. I attribute my staying in good health and healing miracle, to my healing sessions with you, my exercise and nutritional plan.

He did a nutritional program I suggested, using probiotics, vitamins, and compression socks. Some of the herbs and supplements he had been taking heated up his body, so I took him off those. We also changed his routine of exercise to do four or five twenty-minute walks per week, and he is surfing again.

I created a program for him, as I do for all my clients, by combining it with traditional mainstream medicine. I love that combination because it works great. As someone with a career background in mainstream medicine, every day I see the benefits of personalizing treatments based on a client's individual needs, using the best of what both traditional and alternative medicine have to offer.

I do find that, in general, people who have heart disease and related problems with their heart are experiencing a disorder in the feminine energy sensitive left side of the body. That energy with Sean was compromised. He was a sweet, loving man, and I felt like he didn't use his throat chakra a lot, which I find with a lot of people who are having their heart compromised and their arteries clogged. These issues are often found on the left side, the feminine side, of the body. These individuals are often unable to speak their truths. Oftentimes, they are very creative but have a hard time asserting themselves with others. That is a pattern among my clients that I see occurring on the left side of the body.

Sean was also somebody who wanted to be of more service to his community, but he had been too much of a loner to play that role. Now, after working with me, he has joined groups and goes on retreats. He is more spiritually involved now, moving into the 5th Dimensional space.

ROBIN'S CAROTID ARTERY MIRACLE

At a Liphe Center healing clinic in Connecticut, I met Robin, a psychologist in her early sixties, who wanted a medical scan and healing from me. I knew nothing about her. When I started scanning her with my hands across her body, I was blinking on her left carotid artery. I asked her if she had had surgeries before, and she indicated she had a heart attack and had an operation for mitral valve prolapse and a stent had to be inserted.

I asked her to go into the 5th Dimension and accept the Holy Spirit. I put one hand on the left side of her neck, on the carotid artery, and my right hand I placed on her heart as my Guides guided me to do a circular motion, a form of energy surgery that I do. They told me to ask her, "Will you accept the 5th Dimension?" She said yes and exhaled in one long, deep breath. I said Hail Mary three times, and Mother Mary came. She kept breathing out. Three times, she felt the Mother Mary Energy. She looked at me with tears. "You said the Marys in threes." I said yes, and she was sad but happy. "I feel Mary is here." I said she is here. Her neck from the operation was stiff and hard, and it became like silk. She said, "It's gone." She could move her neck easier.

Often, when I do take a dark round negative matter off the carotid artery, I save people from having a heart attack or stroke. I knew the Divine had saved Robin from having another heart attack.

A couple of days later, she wrote to me:

I didn't know what to expect. Kimberly didn't know anything about me. But she found my stent in my neck, I had a blockage a couple of years ago. And the dark energy that's been around that inflammation and down my left side where I've had a lack of circulation over the years and she found problems in my stomach which I had carried for a long time and I didn't even know about that. She found everything that was going on physically. The healing opened me up to blessings of who we really are connected to God, we are one, his will be done. These were healings that took place from God physically, emotionally, and spiritually.

JOAN'S DIABETES MIRACLE

Joan was a filmmaker from Australia, about thirty-five years old, complaining of feeling tired, shaky, and sweaty much of the time. She worked long hours on movie sets and got maybe four hours of sleep a night. "No one can figure out what is wrong with me," she admitted.

She experienced pain on the right side of her body, which is interesting because that's the masculine side, which emphasizes strength, courage, and independence. As I stood over her and started to scan her, waving my hands and feeling my Guides, through my eyes, communicating with me, I knew that she had multiple things going on. I scanned her quickly, with my hands gliding quickly across her body, and I blinked right on her throat. I said, "I know there is something wrong with your thyroid."

Then I went to the back of her head and to the pituitary, and I blinked there. I went down to her kidneys, and I blinked there. "I think there is something wrong with your kidney, your hormones, and your thyroid for sure." I diagnosed her in two minutes.

She was like, "Really!" I said, "Absolutely. I just started working out of my office, but I will retire now if you don't have diabetes and something wrong with your kidneys." This was in 2015, right after I had opened my office to see clients.

I told her she needed to get a blood test to confirm what I found, and when she got the testing done, they found out she was diabetic. This was causing her abnormal thyroid function. That was another example of me working with mainstream medicine, finding out right away whether my initial scanning diagnosis was correct. Sometimes people using only holistic medicine don't want to see someone practicing conventional medicine, but I always urge them to do so in order to confirm my initial scan results.

Joan went many years being misdiagnosed. She had a rare hormone-based form of diabetes. She might get up in the morning and just have a protein shake, then not eat on the movie set until mid-afternoon and then she would eat only a salad without any protein in it. You can't just have fruit in the morning or you are going to crash. It sets you up for diabetes by not having a balanced diet.

If you're going to be vegan or on a solely plant-based diet, you need to consume the right sources of protein. It's important to emphasize that I never recommend eating fish because of the mercury found in most fish, a toxin that triggers neurological disorders.

Joan wrote to me:

> I just wanted to let you know how truly grateful I am for the healing. The pain on the right side of my body has completely dissolved as has the persistent soreness and swelling in my throat. I am sleeping deeply for the first time in many years. I had not been quite right for a long time, though able to work and not horribly ill. I had almost forgotten what it was like to be in complete good health. More than anything I feel like my old self again. You may remember that you identified the pituitary gland as the source of the problem. You were right. I figured out the injury to the top of my head which caused the problem for 11 years. It also explains why my insulin levels were measured as pre-diabetic when my diet and lifestyle is very healthy. No doctor could explain this. It is a type of diabetes called Insipidus, which is rare and related to a deficiency of the pituitary hormone that regulates kidney function. It makes sense as my kidneys are often sore. I was tested

and now I know you were completely correct. I just wanted to let you know how truly impressed I am with the specificity of your diagnosis scanning and the miraculous speed with which you were able to do this.

RALPH'S TYPE 2 DIABETES

My client Ralph, who is in his fifties, had bad eating habits and weight issues and came in for a scan and healing. I didn't know anything about him the first day I met him. He was in the healing community as a crystal store owner.

He lay on my table, very eager for a healing, and he had been to a lot of famous healers. I put rose oil on his third eye and the palms of his hands, and placed the selenite crystals in his palms, and I asked him to enter the 5th Dimension. As I scanned his body, I found a tumor in the right side of his brain, and I blinked on his thyroid, his prostate, and his ankles. When I reviewed the information with him through Spirit, I told him I thought he had a brain tumor and a thyroid or diabetes problem. I thought his ankles were swollen because of diabetes.

Ralph said I was correct, he had both a brain tumor and type 2 diabetes. He also had gout on his right foot for three years. I asked what he had been doing for his diabetes, and he replied that he had been taking a medication but he was still having symptoms. He was worried about the brain tumor because surgery had been recommended to him. He asked what I recommended. At that point, I suggested we do a healing, and then I would go over a treatment plan with him.

I was in a deep trance state, and the Guides asked if we could do a healing on his brain and lay hands on his thyroid. He said yes. I stared at him, and the Guides spoke to him, "You are in the 5th Dimension." He repeated back to me, "I am in the 5th Dimension." I was saying Hail Mary's and he was chanting in Hebrew. He felt a release and began to cry.

After the session, the Guides directed me to write out a four-page treatment plan of supplements and probiotics, I put oxygen therapy on both ankles, and that brought down the swelling on the right ankle. I sat down after each follow-up session and wrote down what the Guides wanted him to do. He felt extremely happy. He followed up with me two months later after an MRI of his brain, which found the tumor had shrunk. He improved his diet by going on a holistic regimen and nutritional plan, and he lost weight as a result.

Ralph completed the entire homework plan I'd given him because he'd become a believer in my mediumship as a result of my Guides' accurate scan. He drinks spring water from glass bottles now, consumes only organic meats, and he goes to the gym five times a week and does yoga. I still see him periodically for checkups, and his diabetes is under control and the tumor has shrunk almost to nothing. It's a Miracle.

CINDY'S THYROID MIRACLE

Cindy was in her fifties when my Guides picked her out of an audience of one hundred or so people at a Conscious Life Expo in Los Angeles. I brought her up on the stage so I could scan her. I found a huge goiter on the right side of her neck. She was having a hard time swallowing. I asked if she wanted a healing, and she said yes.

Some people came up on stage with me to watch as I laid hands on the goiter, and in minutes, it diminished in size by about three or four inches, right there onstage, and we captured that happening on camera. My scan also picked up two thyroid nodes, but I didn't detect any thyroid cancer. After the healing, she exclaimed to the crowd, "It's off my throat. I am so honored that God did this healing for me today." One lady standing nearby put her hand on Cindy's throat and proclaimed to the crowd, "Yes, it's gone!" Everyone cheered and said amen.

The goiter was gone, and Cindy didn't know she had a thyroid problem until I found it with my scan. She contacted me about six months later to say my scan had been correct, diagnostic testing had confirmed she didn't have thyroid cancer. Her thyroid nodes were benign. The problem was that her thyroid wasn't regulating properly.

Her thyroid problem was chronic and could have lasted for years, but it can be controlled with medicines. She also needed to make some lifestyle changes. She was drinking tap water and drinking out of plastic bottles, she had a diet high in sugars, didn't get sufficient sleep, and she had anger issues and yelled at her kids a lot. Drinking out of plastic bottles, using fluoride in toothpaste, and eating high-sugar diets with lots of fruit, these are typical contributing factors to people I have seen with thyroid problems.

Cindy also needs to have more chakra healing to strengthen the feminine side of her body because she speaks—and controls her life—with masculine energy. Femininity in the world right now isn't grounded, which is one reason why I find more problems in the left sides of the bodies of people I scan. We women are in a time period where, in order to be heard, we are forced out of feminine energy.

HEATHER'S LYMPH NODE MIRACLE

Heather had heard about me through a friend who had a successful healing of a breast lump I removed. She also heard me on a nationwide radio show. After having a swollen lymph node on her throat for many years, she came in to experience my healing work.

She came in with an open mind to have a holistic healing experience, though she wasn't a spiritual person and had a conservative banking background. I asked her multiple questions, but nothing regarding her diagnosis. When she lay down on the Reiki bed, I waved my hands over her body and asked her to leave the 3rd Dimension, explaining this is the Dimension where we get sick. I asked her to envision the 5th Dimension, where we can be healed, and see herself floating in an energy of love.

She said she believed in God. She held the selenite crystals, and as I scanned her, I went straight to her body hot spots, which were the thyroid on both sides of her neck, the nodules on her throat, and her breasts. Within three minutes, I knew what was happening to her. She was elated when I told her she had swollen nodes and a hormone imbalance, because she hadn't told me any of this. I counted with my blinks back nineteen or twenty years as being how long she had these conditions, which she affirmed.

She asked me if she could be healed, and I blinked yes. I rubbed my hands together and put the holy water around her throat, at the thyroid. I asked her what she wanted to say as a chant or prayer to release the energy around her throat. She wanted to say the Hail Mary. She stared at me and started reciting the Hail Marys, and as I put my hand on the lump on her neck, it dissolved and just slid off. The Guides then moved my hand to anoint her breast with holy water, rose oil, and olive oil, and I began to remove the cysts as we repeated a mantra together, "I release this negative energy out of my body, out of the room, and out of the Universe, NOW! I am love, I am light, I am in the 5th Dimension. And I am healed."

She sat up, feeling her neck. Again, she looked into my eyes, crying, and was very thankful.

I had two follow-up sessions with Heather. Meantime, she did the protocols in my lifestyle agreement plan and a low-carb, low-sugar diet, and she took the probiotics and supplements I suggested, along with the spring water. She also did chakra-balancing exercises with me, relationship cord–breaking exercises, and breathing exercises to reduce her stress and break old patterns, teaching her how to be in the 5th Dimension. She was successful at that. When she got her next ultrasound results back, the enlarged nodule had gone, eliminating the need for surgery.

Heather began attending my events and made the following statement at a public healing in front of the RA MA Institute in Venice, California:

> For the last twenty-some odd years I have had on the right side of my neck a lymph node that has been bothering me, and every time I got sick, it swelled up more and hit on the outside of my

esophagus. So finally, about a year ago I went to an ENT [ear, nose, and throat] doctor, and he was feeling both of them and he said let's get an ultrasound. So I finally went and had the ultrasound and had no idea the left side of my throat was even more enlarged, the right was nothing, the left one was really enlarged and I can't feel it. I had no idea. So in any case, he just wanted to wait and watch it. I was hoping to get a biopsy, but that's fine. It wasn't meant to be. So I overheard Kimberly on *Fade to Black* radio show with Jimmy Church. I was just so curious I thought, you know what, why does it hurt? I'd rather not have to go through chemo or anything like that, it was not worth the money.

You don't even tell Kimberly what's wrong. I didn't want to tell her, so she could find out on her own, and she did. I am in banking. I have the most conservative lifestyle, you would never believe something like this, it's amazing. She did the body scan, she picked up on the lymph nodes right away, and I didn't say anything. She picked up on my left breast, which had been aching for years, and she found the cysts and released them off my breast. I sat up and she said, "Okay, feel your neck." I felt my neck and said, "They are gone."

SHEILA'S HORMONAL MIRACLE

Having a hormone imbalance is common among my clients, affecting about 60 percent of the women and men I see. It's also common among young girls if they miss a period and a doctor puts them on medications. A concussion can cause a hormonal imbalance, as can types 1 and 2 diabetes, extreme chronic stress, hyperglycemia, and an underactive or overactive thyroid. Men also experience too much or too little testosterone.

Thirty-two-year-old Sheila, a corporate management employee, saw me after she had been trying to get pregnant for a year and a half and failed, even though she took fertility drugs. Her doctors couldn't figure out why. I knew she had a hormonal imbalance when I first scanned her. Way before she had first tried to get pregnant, she had been suffering from an undiagnosed hormonal imbalance in the aftermath of having had a concussion. Added to that, she and her husband were stressed out over trying for more than a year to conceive a child.

Where my scans generally find hormonal imbalances in the pituitary and other regions of the brain, the back of the neck (the T1) and of course, the thyroid gland. And sometimes I will detect hormonal imbalance in the pancreas. When I get the hot flashes during scanning, as it happens when I detect cancer, it's a different kind of hot flash. I get a different type of blinking. When I get six blinks, I know that's about the hormones, while with cancer, I get more hot flashes. For hormonal imbalances, I just get right eye blinks.

A lot of times, I can see the imbalance in their left eye, in their cornea, their left eye is weak. Sometimes they have a problem with their left eye, which can be because of their blood pressure being off. Hormonal issues can also be caused by inflammatory issues, which can be connected to the gut. Most people with hormonal problems have gut issues or urinary tract issues. It's all connected.

She was having hot flashes, so I put her on a supplement program, including herbs that I like to work with, and this helped her to produce good eggs. I got her off plastics and into clean water. When she went in for in vitro fertilization, which would have cost her $20,000, they said, "You don't need it. You're pregnant."

You would be surprised how many people have had head injuries that resulted in hormone imbalances. They also have extremely high toxicity levels in their body. A lot of women with hormone imbalances have had their uteruses taken out and are on bioidentical hormones, and they're eating high doses of fish, particularly sushi. The next step for them could be hormone imbalance or cancer because of the high mercury and estrogen content now found in most fish.

An energetic pattern I've seen with hormone imbalances is that often there is some grieving having to do with their relationship with a parent. I do a prayer breaking the energetic cord between them and their parents, or whoever raised them, and who may have hurt them energetically in the past. It doesn't necessarily have to be their parents. It could be anyone who has hurt them.

AMY'S ADRENAL FATIGUE MIRACLE

Amy came into my office with her mom, exhibiting a range of symptoms. She was in her early twenties, an avid long-distance runner who had just gotten out of college and aspired to be a professional athlete. Her mom was worried about her because she felt constantly fatigued and dizzy, with extreme anxiety and irregular bowel movements and menstrual cycles. When she would get up in the morning, she felt complete exhaustion and could no longer exercise. Her eyes looked withdrawn, she had no appetite, and she felt like she was in a mental fog and going crazy. This had been going on for six months.

When Amy got on the table, I started scanning with both my hands, and my blinking went right to her adrenal glands, finding them swollen. Our adrenal glands are triangular-shaped and located above both kidneys, functioning as part of our endocrine system. I also blinked negative on her thyroid area. I pressed down on an adrenal gland, and she reacted painfully. High degrees of stress can trigger adrenal fatigue, and Amy had put intense pressure on herself to become a major athlete. That raised her cortisol levels, and over time, it had exhausted her.

I felt she was going through adrenal fatigue (she didn't have any idea that was the name of the condition) but her symptoms matched what she had. But when I explained it was a hormonal imbalance, both Amy and her mother expressed the feeling this was true. Amy wanted a healing, so I placed both my hands into her adrenal area and we went into prayer, and my Guides and I guided her into the 5th Dimension. As I moved my hands in a circle, she chanted Om. Once the healing was over, she said the pain had disappeared from her adrenal area. She felt amazing. It was miraculous. They both were overjoyed and so happy.

I immediately put her on a low-sugar diet and a regimen of probiotics and supplements. She saw me three more times and made complete lifestyle adjustments to relieve stress. She moved out from her mom's house and got a roommate, and that eliminated some stress emanating from her mother's desire for her to succeed as an athlete. She went gluten-free and cut out alcohol, dairy, sugar, and all inflammatory foods. Her digestive issues went away, as did her headaches, and she once again looked amazing, glowing, and without any depression. She continued doing her chanting and prayers with my 5th Dimensional CD that I gave her. This transformation occurred over a period of six months until all her adrenal fatigue symptoms disappeared. By being super busy all the time, we run the risk of having adrenal fatigue, a burnout condition that can develop into even worse conditions. When it happens, you're getting a warning you need to act as soon as symptoms occur.

Adrenal fatigue is a condition that undermines the immune system if left unchecked. With Amy's story, it is reassuring to know that when you have these symptoms, you can heal in the 5th Dimension by making lifestyle changes.

In my alternative practice, I have found that many hormonal issues and problems link back to diet and the use of bioidentical hormones, including estrogen and progesterone. While I realize that the prescription of bioidentical hormones is standard practice in Western medicine these days, I have seen more harm done than good. I have found that for most of my clients with healthy diets, their hormones can be balanced through natural foods.

I encourage all who suspect the possibility of a hormone imbalance to see their health care practitioners to have their hormone levels checked. Those with hormone imbalances should carefully evaluate all their options before putting anything into their bodies. I take a very conservative approach on taking herbs for hormonal imbalances because some herbs can have the propensity to thin the blood—especially in cases of hormonal endometriosis and ovarian cancers.

Amy did her two follow-up sessions with me through Skype. I did my routine medical intuitive health scan over the computer screen as she easily went into the 5th Dimension. I did not pick up on any lower abdominal issues or immune issues. We have continued to work together on balancing her chakras and keeping her throat chakra clear. This is wonderful for her and helped her find balance. Amy is now back to running, and she feels much better. Amy remains grateful for my Guide's teachings about the 5th Dimension.

JEANETTE'S COVID-19 VIRUS MIRACLE

During the first month of the 2020 COVID-19 pandemic, Jeanette signed up for a virtual Skype session with me. She was sixty-five years old, an accountant staying at home in quarantine. She had heard about me through Dr. Joe Dispenza and wanted me to conduct a medical intuitive scan and healing. She was feeling very anxious and felt she needed the scan right away.

When I got online with her, I explained the process step by step. I asked her to stand back from her computer screen so I could see her entire body, then I asked her to take three or four deep breaths, and open her hands fully to her side, palms out, like the wings of an Angel, as she recited the chant, "I am love, I am light."

I waved my hand over her body, from the top of her head down to her feet. I got immediate download information from my Guides about her condition and saw a blueprint from her going directly to her right lung. I sensed she might have the coronavirus. I did both a front and back scan, a 360-degree view of her, and received hot flashes almost immediately, getting three hits on her—on her uterus, her right lung, and her throat. She confirmed it as true each time.

She began having difficulty breathing about five minutes into the scan, so I asked her to sit down.

"I'll tell you what my Guides are picking up. They're telling me your right lung is weak, and your esophagus is in some difficulty. Your uterus and bladder have had dysfunction issues." She said I was correct on all counts. She said her uterus had been taken out.

"Have you been diagnosed with the coronavirus?" I asked her.

She said yes.

"My Guides are telling me your right lung is weak." She confirmed that her right lung was collapsing and she was on an inhaler.

People who get the virus, and end up with the severest symptoms, often are immune suppressed and suffering emotional traumas. In Jeanette's case, she was only having coffee and a banana in the mornings, and a shake for lunch. She was deprived of proper nutrition, and she was drinking tap water. She had also been suffering from depression after her husband had cheated on her and abused her.

She was dumbfounded when the Guides told me about her uterus problems. She had undergone a C-section, multiple fibroids, a leaky bladder, and her immune system had crashed, all a decade earlier. I think that was why she got susceptible to the coronavirus—a combination of a weakened immune system, a hormone imbalance, and too much stress. She believed she had contracted the virus from a baseball event she attended with her grandkids. She couldn't get rid of the cough, because the virus was stuck in her right lung.

She wasn't religious, but I chose to call in the Holy Spirit, and we entered the 5th Dimension together.

"I am in the 5th Dimension, I am love, I am love, I am light," we chanted together. She rubbed her hands together, as I directed her to. She went into the 5th Dimension very easily, feeling a tingling sensation in her hands. I had her place her hands around her throat and say, "I release any negative energy off my throat."

I had her follow the movement of my hands, being directed by my Guides, continuing to remove the negative energy off her throat and then off her lung, followed by her uterus. She did this three times: "I release the negative energy off my uterus, NOW. I release the negative energy off my bladder, NOW. I release the negative energy off my lungs, NOW."

On the third repetition, she started to cough up phlegm, and she felt a release. She said chills went through her body and her breathing improved.

She had demonstrated full trust in me. This threw her into the full belief that accompanies an Awakening.

"Whatever you have for me, I will do," she vowed.

She was willing and ready, after just one session, to change her diet and take the supplements I recommended. I asked her to tell me in detail about her diet. She had been taking high doses of turmeric and apple cider vinegar, which I suggested she discontinue because they were heating up her body. She was eating only fruit in the morning and shakes throughout the day, some chicken and white rice, followed by intermittent fasting. That was her diet for the previous three months. I don't recommend eating chicken or fish, and she agreed to give up both.

I put her on an immune-boosting, high-oxygen diet, eating small meals throughout the day, with lots of hydration, and a probiotic with the Solgar vitamins. She needed someone patting her on the back to help break up the phlegm, the mucus collecting in her lungs. But living alone, she needed to lie flat on the floor, doing breathing techniques using an incentive spirometer to build up her lung strength.

When I rescanned her at the end of our session, I had her raise her hands up and say, "I am healed. Amen."

All of us live in a time of uncertainty and fear about both the known and unknown viruses that lurk around us, the COVID-19 virus being just the most recent disrupter of our lives.

We have the capacity and the knowledge to take the steps necessary to protect ourselves and our loved ones. These commonsense steps begin with keeping our immune systems strong, since immunity is our first line of defense against the entire range of viruses threatening us.

Regardless of your age, your sex, or state of your health, everyone can benefit from boosting their immune system to help prevent, treat, or recover from viral onslaughts and the effects of toxins in the environment. Microbes are getting stronger and stronger, and our antibiotics and other drugs are failing to adequately control them. That puts even more pressure on us individually to adopt healthy lifestyles that help protect our immunity.

I have witnessed firsthand the remarkable recoveries that can occur when the immune system is strengthened, so I am a firm believer that by combining practical tips to boost your immune system with a consciousness rooted in 5th Dimension teachings and self-healing principles, you will help protect yourself and others from health impairments.

We are doing what we can to move into a better place. We know we must send love into the world, and this is imperative, because we know we are powerful and love is the real source of trusting our highest path of believing in the Miracles of healing. We can all rise together to make this happen.

PETER'S CHRONIC VIRAL CONDITION—SHINGLES

Peter had heard of me from listening to my weekly radio show. He was in his fifties and had a complete immune system crash, developing non-Hodgkin's lymphoma. When he came in with his girlfriend to see me, he was having difficulty breathing (he brought his oxygen tank with him) and had gone through traditional chemotherapy trials, yet his condition seemed to be getting worse. In fact, he had been told he had only a few months to live.

He wanted to explain what was wrong with him before I scanned him. He was a gentle and spiritual man and quickly entered the 5th Dimension with me as I started blinking around his eyes and lips, his lower back, and his spine. I told him something was going on in his eyes, and he said, "I have shingles in my eyes and in my spine, and I am in a lot of pain." He confirmed my scanning that he had shingles in his mouth and throat.

Once shingles gets into your nerves and spinal cord, you are in excruciating pain. The only real treatment is to boost your immune system. Numerous scientific studies show a link between having cancer and your risk of developing shingles, which may have been what triggered Peter's serious and painful case of shingles, a disease in the herpes family that further depletes the immune system.

When I scan someone and get a hit on shingles, I get blinking on their spinal cord or their eyes and lips. With shingles, if you have an outbreak, it can go into your brain, and you can get neuropathy, losing the ability to walk. It usually affects one side of the body, and in Peter's case, it was the left side.

We did prayers and chants and healing sessions together. He had been searching for spiritual answers by living in an ashram and following the teachings of Yogananda, so he was quite open and ready for healings from the masters.

I got him on my regimen of supplements. He stopped using the Rife machine, which produces low-energy waves that some alternative medicine practitioners prescribe as a cancer treatment, even though it isn't FDA approved. I didn't see any positive results for him from using it.

He was an intense case because he seemed like a dead man walking. The shingles were inside the lids of his eyes. I had gloves on and couldn't touch his eyes. I used my special blessed ormus cream around the sides of his eyes and on his spine, and he did 108 rounds of chants and prayers to the music he brought in. (Ormus cream is a solution of alchemically activated sea minerals that reduces inflammation and expedites the healing process.)

He continued working with me for six months. He didn't have an appetite when I first met him, but during his work with me, he started eating again and developed an even stronger faith. I suggested he stay away from sugars and high-carb diets like pastas. Lysine is a supplement I recommended because it has been an effective treatment for a range of viruses. I often suggest 1,500 mg of lysine a day to people without shingles, but my Guides say to double that for people who have the disease. Lysine builds up immune support—foods high in lysine include turkey, beef, and eggs—so it can also be taken as a preventative. The most you should take is about 3,000 mg a day, and I suggest using Solgar, the most powerful lysine brand supplement I know. (I do not profit from its sale.)

I also put him on holistic GABA as a painkiller, green tea as an antioxidant, and the herb echinacea for his immune system support. (GABA is a natural brain neurotransmitter that also dissolves anxiety and improves sleep.)

Peter and his girlfriend moved to Arizona because his oncologist had a new program that was based in a residential hospital there, where his girlfriend also lived, and he wanted to be near her. He asked my thoughts about leaving my office sessions, and I said we could continue our healing health scans and programs on Skype, and with the alternative care, nothing should change. He was very excited to leave Los Angeles. He has continued to improve and keeps in touch with me through our Skype healings, which include praying in the 5th Dimension, walking him through the step-by-step release of blocks of energy, and gathering a clear focus to stay in the frequency with GOD. This helps him with his chemo and understanding this is a constant daily practice. The laughter and the chants bring healing into his heart chakras as he listens to my meditation CDs. It helps uplift him during his chemo infusions. He looks better and better. Peter is a warrior, and his girlfriend reports he is truly in recovery.

People who get viral infections often had previously weakened their immune systems in various ways, such as receiving treatment for cancer. With any viral infections, you have to lay off the sugar. That includes consuming alcohol, since it is converted into sugar by the body.

Sometimes clients ask my Guides, "How many drinks can I have? One drink a night? One drink a week?" I ask my clients in turn, "What are you really willing to let go in your life if you want to have a clean diet and heal?" Sometimes the Guides will say, just drink twice a week, but sometimes they will say nothing. It's not forever.

A lot of people say they are a vegan or a vegetarian, but at night, the real truth is revealed . . . they're regularly eating Häagen-Dazs ice cream, or some other non-vegan or non-vegetarian item.

It's time to be truthful and to go all the way, cleaning up your diet *and* your relationship to the truth. You have to walk the talk if you want to be healed and stay healed.

APPENDIX 3

Scientific and Medical Evaluations of Kimberly's Abilities

C. Norman Shealy, M.D., Ph.D., a neurosurgeon and psychologist, who helped launch the career of medical intuitive Caroline Myss, described his work studying the intuitive medical diagnosis and healing abilities of Kimberly Meredith in a 2018 YouTube video (https://www.youtube.com/watch?v=Ntji4_HiLMk):

> I am Dr. Norman Shealy. I am the CEO and founder of the American Holistic Medicine Association. For the last forty-five years, I've had the pleasure of working with a number of talented spiritual healers, starting with Olga Worrall, the most studied healer in history. Since that time, I have done a total of two hundred different patients with a variety of healers, perhaps six altogether. The most interesting thing to me about spiritual healing from a physical point of view is that they can change an electroencephalogram from a distance of up to one thousand miles, within seconds. So my standard test, other than looking at the possibility of healing, is to see whether the healer can affect the EEG from some distance. It doesn't seem to make any difference whether they are outside the room or miles away.

This week, I've had the pleasure of working with Kimberly Meredith. She is the most unusual of all these healers. She does much more hands-on work, both in making the diagnosis, and she is very accurate in picking up exactly where there is pathology or symptoms of pathology. Today, in addition to working with the eighteenth patient that we've worked with together, I asked her to do an EEG on one of the patients. So the patient is in the room, with the computerized EEG hooked up, the patient lies there for twelve minutes for a baseline of what's going on in her brain in deep relaxation. Then for the next twelve minutes, Kimberly, outside the room, maybe fifteen feet away at the most, but through the wall is sending healing. The EEG on this woman, when she was at rest, was in delta, deep relaxation, one to three cycles per second, fairly strong. Interestingly, during the twelve minutes that Kimberly was sending healing, the brain just became quiet. The delta disappeared, and there was no other frequency there. Just one tiny little spot on the back part of the brain, on the right [the visual center], as if she was just on the verge of going to sleep. The difference was quite striking. There was no question that it changed abruptly, and to me, this shows that Kimberly is, among other things, almost certainly focusing scalar energy. I don't know of anything else that could travel through a wall that fast except scalar energy. It doesn't matter. What matters is this proves she is having a physiological change on the patient. That was as good a change as you will ever see.

See also: New Realities 2018 video interview with Dr. Norm Shealy and Kimberly Meredith (https://www.youtube.com/watch?v =ZnNcwI-NLjM).

Interview excerpts with Dr. Shealy speaking about his tests on Kimberly Meredith's medical intuitive skills and healing abilities:

She is extremely accurate in picking up where there are disturbances anywhere in the body, from the brain to the toes.

She scans the body and then says, "There is something wrong here, this is okay, there is something wrong here." Then she goes back and does it a second time and begins to home in on what it is, what is exactly wrong and what organ is involved. I've worked with lots of healers, and I've never seen a healer do it that way. Most healers don't make that much of a diagnosis.

She touches [the body], while she is doing the diagnosis, so to speak, and then when she begins to treat, she presses very hard into the area and may knead and roll that area, sometimes for several minutes. She has the patient breathe very deeply, and she asks the patient, at some point, I believe in the Holy Spirit and through the Holy Spirit, I am healing. The results are almost instantaneous. The patients feel none or much less pain and more mobility. The difference with Kimberly is, the average healer barely touches the patient. She both diagnoses and then she treats, which is very different from most medical intuitives.

OTHER SCIENTIFIC EVALUATIONS

Psy-Tek Labs, Encinitas, California

Under the supervision of research director Gaetan Chevalier, Ph.D., an engineering physicist, Kimberly's abilities were tested in 2017 as part of the Psy-Tek Subtle Energy Lab ongoing subtle energies (energy medicine) research program.

Wrote Chevalier, after examining thermography images of a patient's knees, before and after Kimberly's healing treatment:

It is clear that there is a decrease in inflammation in the anterior part of the right leg, a few inches below the knee two days after your treatment. These images also show a decrease in inflammation of the lateral side of the right leg a few inches below the knee.

From the healing I have seen at the Conscious Life Expo (I was at your presentation when you worked on a lady [who] was in extreme pain and in bad shape overall) and the improvements we have seen in our lab, it is clear that you have genuine healing abilities.

IONS—Institute of Noetic Sciences—Petaluma, California

From April 6 to 12, 2019, Kimberly Meredith was the subject of an ongoing pilot study of mediumship and healing abilities called the Exceptional Healers Pilot Study, at the science research lab of the Institute of Noetic Sciences (IONS), founded by the late NASA astronaut and moonwalker Dr. Edgar Mitchell.

Said lead study scientist Garret Yount, Ph.D.: "We were indeed privileged to be able to have Kimberly Meredith participate in our Exceptional Healers Pilot Study being conducted at IONS. We spent a wonderful collaborative week together. She was one of the exceptional healers in our study. We would like to do a further study designed to focus only on her unique talents."

Overall preliminary results of the 2019 IONS Exceptional Healers Pilot Study are as follows:

The scale of this study was significant relative to previous studies of energy medicines—nearly 200 individual healing sessions from 17 different practitioners and their unique modalities across nine months. As a pilot study, we were seeking a number of proofs of feasibility that would allow us to develop a standardized suite of subjective and objective measures for the rigorous exploration of energy healing.

These early and important proofs include:

Clinical significance in pain reduction: The gold standard of any healing process is to achieve clinical significance—that the treatments result in real, genuine, and noticeable effects on daily life. This was achieved.

In focusing on carpal tunnel pain, we were able to verifiably achieve this important milestone of providing people immediate and lasting relief. This was a necessary foundation for bringing energy healing into the lab and creating objective conditions for studying real-world impact.

Measurable effects on H-O bonds in water and Quantum Noise Generator (QNG): Our preliminary conclusion of the analyses is that it appears as though the healing sessions caused entropic ripples in spacetime. From this pilot study, we do not yet know the cause of these effects, but we have verified that the subjective experiences of pain reduction are being backed up by objective data. Water samples during healing sessions absorbed more infrared energy, suggesting the H-O bond was stretched and utilizing a QNG we detected notable deviations in background entropy, all pointing to a clear "disturbance in the force."

While this pilot study was not powered to definitively test hypotheses, some of the measures yielded provocative results. We are ready to move from a pilot study to a more targeted formal study, and get that much closer to the normalization of energy medicine in healing pain, both temporary and chronic.

TESTIMONIALS FROM HEALTH CARE PROFESSIONALS

"In the world of alternative, holistic, energy medicine, Kimberly is the real deal. Kimberly is the most gifted medical intuitive I know.

Her ability to tap into the body and determine abnormalities is unlike anything I have experienced before. During my personal healing sessions, I witnessed her clear connection with the Divine. I felt a sense of calm and that we were surrounded by Angelic energies. I could feel the energetic shifts that were happening in different areas of my body as Kimberly worked on them. She intuitively knew the exact areas of disharmony in my body. After my sessions I noticed a significant and permanent improvement not just physically, but mentally and spiritually as well. This world is blessed to have such a wonderfully gifted person like Kimberly, who has committed her life to sharing her unique abilities to assist those in need. I highly recommend my family, friends and patients to see her."—Michael F. MacDonald, M.D., Detroit, Michigan, American Board of Urology

"I have been in healthcare for fifty years, including research, hospital, laboratory, and private settings. I have seen many healings, by many different means. Frankly, not only do I feel much better after Kimberly Meredith's healing session, but she has a powerful uplifting presence that is quite unique and exceptional. Thank you, Kimberly, for your extraordinary gifts and your willingness to help others."— Ronald Drucker, M.D., Pembroke Pines, Florida

"I have been working with my client Barbara for some time as a physical therapist. It was really amazing visually to see her upper arm because the tissue itself wasn't so poignant and was completely flattened (after the session with Kimberly) and when I palpated it, the adhesions that had been in there were completely different, it was flatter, and some of the knots that were palpable in the upper arm were completely gone. It was a really beautiful thing to observe and very exciting for Barbara to experience the healing."—Jeanne Morgante, doctor of physical therapy

"I am a two-time cancer survivor. I am a licensed marriage and family therapist from Sunnyvale, California. I first witnessed Kimberly

Meredith at the 2018 New Living Expo. I saw Kimberly scanning and healing others with cancer. It inspired me to have a medical intuitive scan in which Kimberly discovered and dissolved a tumor in my right breast. She also found in my left breast a tumor and she discovered and removed many post-cancerous residual hard lumps from two past surgeries which I had never told her about. Kimberly also healed and smoothed the entire incision with her hands."—La Von Bobo, MS, LMFT, CST, El Camino, California

"I'm sending a long-overdue thank-you for our session and your time, energy, attention, and thoughtfulness. Your medical intuitive scan was very accurate. I've been using the Ormus cream, and residing in a space of gratitude navigating everything moving forward (and eating more protein and following your daily suggestions). I look forward to crossing paths again. Much gratitude."—Felicia Tomasko, RN, author, *LA Yoga* magazine

"Thank you so very much for your medical intuitive body scan. The accuracy was amazing and the healing session. Thank you for your loving kindness and generosity!! I loved seeing you work and feeling the healing energy! The lymph node on my left neck area is completely gone now, and I feel so much better. I so appreciate all you do for others, and words can't express my gratitude for your session!"—Dr. Michelle Cohen, licensed clinical psychologist, host of *LA Talk Radio*

ACKNOWLEDGMENTS

The Guides and I were honored and extremely grateful to write this book. I am so excited that I can finally present the finished work to you, at what feels like the perfect time in our evolution and Ascension. Throughout the process, blessings and encouragement have come from many sources. First of all, I would like to express my deepest respect for my beautiful and inspiring sister Kelly Zalba. Thank you for your love and support—I love and appreciate you so much.

Writing this book has been a profound experience and also a fun and exciting one with the Guides. Without the assistance of my literary agent, Bill Gladstone of Waterside Productions, and my publisher, Joel Fotinos of St. Martin's Essentials, the book you are reading would not have come into being. I'm deeply grateful for Joel and Bill's guidance, for this book is helpful to the readers because of the creative process.

Just as I am a 5th Dimensional Medium healer helping my clients achieve optimal health, I believe they are 5th Dimensional editors and publishing advisers able to use their energies to assist in this beautiful manuscript.

I also want to acknowledge my editorial adviser Randall Fitzgerald. Randall spent hours helping me refine early drafts of the manuscript. Thank you, Randall, for staying on task throughout the process with the Guides.

The following people have provided enormous encouragement and have witnessed the 5th Dimensional Miracles with me. You have contributed to my growth as a Medium and healer along my journey. My heart is filled with so much gratitude for you—you mean the world to me! Thank you.

Dr. C. Norman Shealy, Robert Hayhurst, Alan Steinfeld, Saige Walker, Medium Thomas John, James Carmen, Robert Quicksilver, Eric Middleman, Wendy Zahler, Devon Blaine, Gary Garver, Trevor Lissauer, Dawna Shuman, Denman Wall, Sandy Manuel, Bridgette Buckley, Jonny Podell, Gwen Hawkes, Josh Freel, Lisa Najjar, Jackie Lappin, Ken Kaufman, Mark Becker, Kenji Kumara, Sam Kiwasz, David Wolfe, Paul Selig, Diana Maxwell, Steven Halpern, Tee Celise, George Sobel, Robin Lerner, Wendy Zahler, Dr. Alex Hakim, Lisa Garr, Pierre Gatling, Carter Mason, Joe Gonzales, Todd Feder, Barbara Silver Slaine, Dannion Brinkley, Wynn Free, Terry Brown, Iris Braydon, Angela Hartman, Tony Camacho, Gail Gladstone, Ryan MacMillan, Steven Dempsey, Thomas Calannio, Katherine Williams, Cassandra Vieten, Dean Radin, Garret Yount, Helané Wahbeh, Margaret McCormick, Nancy Thompson, John Zalba, Jeremy C. Gilbreath, and Catherine Oxenberg.

I am filled with gratitude to God, for the guidance to write this important book with its timely messages for all. Finally, heartfelt thanks to my precious "soul family"—my spiritual family members reuniting here on Earth as we learn, grow, and complete our individual missions. You know who you are, and we come into each other's lives for a reason. I have been so fortunate to meet you along the way—may the force be with you!

ABOUT THE AUTHOR

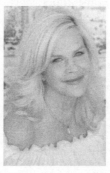

Paul Smith Photography

Kimberly Meredith is a world-renowned medical Medium, trance channeler, hands-on healer, and spiritual teacher. She had two near-death experiences, leaving her in a wheelchair for a year, and through God and the Holy Spirit, she was healed and given the gift of communicating with God through her eyes.

Blessed with a unique array of extraordinary healing and psychic abilities, Kimberly Meredith is quickly gaining recognition as one of the world's most gifted medical mediumship healers and spiritual speakers. Kimberly is a vessel for God, Mother Mary, Ascended Masters, Angels, and advanced civilizations. Kimberly is often compared to Edgar Cayce, the father of holistic medicine, himself a medical

Medium, and the most documented psychic of the twentieth century.

A healer like no other, she bridges the gap between God and science. Kimberly's gifts manifest through blinking up to twenty multidimensional codes, including three consecutive blinks, which indicate Divine Confirmation. She communicates through Divinely guided sign language, and she also speaks in 5th Dimensional Etheric Angelic Light Language in order to heal, awaken, and move humanity forward. Through her healing mediumship and blinking, Kimberly is guided to perform the laying on of hands or psychic surgery. Kimberly has healed and helped many thousands of people, removing tumors, restoring hearing, curing cancer, correcting immobility, and completely ridding people of rare diseases and emotional traumas. She scans the body faster and more accurately than any MRI, ultrasound, or thermography machine, accurately diagnosing diseases and symptoms. She then heals these conditions through the power of the Holy Spirit.

To scientifically prove her abilities, Kimberly has been rigorously tested by numerous highly regarded scientific laboratories, such as the Institute of Noetic Sciences, Psy-Tek Labs, and Dr. Norman Shealy of the American Holistic Medicine Association, all of which validated her extraordinary healing powers, which are measurable even through solid walls. The results were profound. Dr. Shealy's tests of Kimberly recorded her ability to heal even through walls. Dr. Shealy concluded that Kimberly appears to emit scalar energy, a unique type of energy associated with genius inventor Nikola Tesla. In 2017, Kimberly was selected by Psy-Tek Subtle Energy Laboratory and Research Facility to undergo ongoing tests to further understand the inner workings of her talents. In 2019, Kimberly was invited to be tested at the famed IONS Institute of Noetic Sciences, founded by Apollo astronaut Edgar Mitchell, with one of the eminent scientists being Dr. Dean Radin. After participating in multiple double-blind scientific studies, Kimberly's healing abilities are beginning to reveal the convergence of God, Spirituality, and science.

Kimberly leads miraculous worldwide healing events during which many are healed. She has received extensive media attention, including several cover feature appearances, in publications like *LA Yoga* magazine, *Radiance* magazine, *Awareness* magazine, *Whole Life Times* magazine, *The Life Connection Magazine*, Thrive Global, the *New York Daily News*, and *Newlife* magazine.

Kimberly heals people one-on-one, remotely over Skype, and in large group events and expos where she is a featured presenter. Kimberly is a frequent guest on numerous nationally syndicated radio shows and podcasts, where she demonstrates her medical mediumship and healing for people around the world. Many have been healed simply by listening to the sound of her voice.

Kimberly also hosts her own syndicated radio program, *The Medical Intuitive Miracle Show*, broadcast live weekly for two years on KCAA Radio 1050 AM, 102.3 FM, and 106.5 FM, and streaming worldwide on KCAARadio.com, Spotify, Stitcher, iHeartRadio, Tiki, and Speaker.

For more information, visit Kimberly's website at www .thehealingtrilogy.com.

Follow Kimberly on Instagram (www.instagram.com

/meredith.kimberly), Facebook (www.facebook.com/kimberly meredith11/), and Twitter (www.twitter.com/HealingTrilogy).

Visit Kimberly's YouTube channel (to witness 5th Dimensional testimonials and healing) at www.YouTube.com/c/KimberlyMeredithChannelstheHolySpirit.

Sign up for, and read, *The Healing Trilogy Newsletter* at www.thehealingtrilogy.com.

JOIN KIMBERLY MEREDITH'S ANGEL CLUB!

Kimberly's Angel Club membership offers access to a full range of unique extras, bonuses, and opportunities, including special events, online webinar retreats, and unique channeled messages. Angel Club members also get exclusive access to more advanced levels of spiritual instruction on 5th and 12th Dimensional healing, plus additional helpful tools to shield yourself against spiritual warfare.

You also get instant access to Kimberly's Video on Demand Library, where you can view and review events. Plus you get a variety of special offers, opportunities, and exclusive members-only videos and content.

For more information, go to www.thehealingtrilogy .com/angel-club/.

Visit the Healing Trilogy store for healing and meditation audio downloads at https://www .thehealingtrilogy.com/store/.

Sign up for our email list for all of our current events, expos, workshops, and tours. You'll also receive a monthly newsletter. For signing up, you will receive a free video from the Angel Club workshop to view: www.thehealingtrilogy.com.

THE 5TH DIMENSION MORNING HEALING PRAYER

Good morning, Creator,
Good morning, Angels.
Please stay with me,
today and every day,
wherever I go.
Please give me strength,
today and every day,
whatever I do.
Let me have no danger,
today and every day,
whatever I face.
Today and every day,
let no task
overcome me.
Today and every day,
let no trial
overcome my heart.
Today and every day,
I am in the 5th Dimension!
My consciousness
is strong,
my energy
and my mind
are healthy!
I shall have courage,
whatever my day
shall bring.
My protection shield
is made of Christ light!
I know my Divine mission.
I am in the 5th Dimension!
Amen.